Giuliana Scarpati
Ilaria Russo
Annunziata Armenante

Lost in Translation

AF138229

Giuliana Scarpati
Ilaria Russo
Annunziata Armenante

Lost in Translation

Bases of translational medicine

LAP LAMBERT Academic Publishing

Impressum / Imprint

Bibliografische Information der Deutschen Nationalbibliothek: Die Deutsche Nationalbibliothek verzeichnet diese Publikation in der Deutschen Nationalbibliografie; detaillierte bibliografische Daten sind im Internet über http://dnb.d-nb.de abrufbar.

Alle in diesem Buch genannten Marken und Produktnamen unterliegen warenzeichen-, marken- oder patentrechtlichem Schutz bzw. sind Warenzeichen oder eingetragene Warenzeichen der jeweiligen Inhaber. Die Wiedergabe von Marken, Produktnamen, Gebrauchsnamen, Handelsnamen, Warenbezeichnungen u.s.w. in diesem Werk berechtigt auch ohne besondere Kennzeichnung nicht zu der Annahme, dass solche Namen im Sinne der Warenzeichen- und Markenschutzgesetzgebung als frei zu betrachten wären und daher von jedermann benutzt werden dürften.

Bibliographic information published by the Deutsche Nationalbibliothek: The Deutsche Nationalbibliothek lists this publication in the Deutsche Nationalbibliografie; detailed bibliographic data are available in the Internet at http://dnb.d-nb.de.

Any brand names and product names mentioned in this book are subject to trademark, brand or patent protection and are trademarks or registered trademarks of their respective holders. The use of brand names, product names, common names, trade names, product descriptions etc. even without a particular marking in this work is in no way to be construed to mean that such names may be regarded as unrestricted in respect of trademark and brand protection legislation and could thus be used by anyone.

Coverbild / Cover image: www.ingimage.com

Verlag / Publisher:
LAP LAMBERT Academic Publishing
ist ein Imprint der / is a trademark of
OmniScriptum GmbH & Co. KG
Heinrich-Böcking-Str. 6-8, 66121 Saarbrücken, Deutschland / Germany
Email: info@lap-publishing.com

Herstellung: siehe letzte Seite /
Printed at: see last page
ISBN: 978-3-659-69417-2

Copyright © 2015 OmniScriptum GmbH & Co. KG
Alle Rechte vorbehalten. / All rights reserved. Saarbrücken 2015

CHAPTER I

Introduction to Translational Medicine

1.1 Introduction

Translational medicine is the base of biomedicine that promotes the value of investments and actualize the very revolution in modern science. The "bench to bedside synthesizes the role of translational medicine. This part of science is the integrated application of innovative biomarkers, clinical methods, clinical technologies and study designs to improve disease understanding, confidence in human new drug targets and increase confidence in drug candidates. There are many definition about this area of medicine. To understand the translation medicine we should imagine a big puzzle of different area of science, from the engineering to medicine, through the biology. Translational research has different objectives: for example the promotion of benefits for patients and support of investments placed by the private and public sector in biomedical research. It's important underline that the translational medicine research encompasses a complexity of scientific, financial, ethical, regulatory, legislative and practical hurdles that need to be addressed at several levels to make the process efficient. It's provides the knowledge necessary to draw important conclusions from clinical testing regarding disease and the viability of novel drug mechanisms, and represents the instrument of very change that could link the Academy and the Industries for the realization of technology transfer.

1.2 Definition of translational Medicine

Definition of translational medicine is not simple: there are many different considerations about this issue derived from many areas of medicine implicated in the discussion. The term "translational research" appeared as early as 1993, there were relatively few references to this term in the medical literature during the 1990s, and most references were to research about study of cancer. Translational research (TR) is a relatively new area of investigation that ideally involves the integrated application of innovative technologies that include several disciplines including physiology, pathophysiology, natural history of disease, genetics, and proof-of-concept studies of drugs and devices (1). Translational medicine is the integrated application of innovative pharmacology tools, biomarkers, clinical methods, clinical technologies and study designs to improve disease understanding, confidence in human drug targets and increase confidence in drug candidates, understand the therapeutic index in humans, enhance cost-effective decision making in exploratory development and increase phase II success (2).

In the past years we collected commentaries and descriptions about Translational Medicine to stimulate discussion and better understand what Translational Medicine is (3).

"Translational medicine" is not a traditional discipline. It has, however, become a very popular phrase which is being widely used in variable contexts both by the pharmaceutical industry and by academics. The idea of translational medicine is both obvious and persuasive if applied to grant applications to industry of tools of operation. Translational research is one of the most important activities of translational medicine as it supports predictions about probable drug activities across species and is especially important when compounds with unprecedented drug targets are brought to humans for the first time (4). Translational Medicine should be regarded as a two-way road: Bench-to-Bedside and Bedside-to-Bench, to complement testing of novel therapeutic strategies in humans with feedback understanding of how they respond to them. It is, therefore, critical and important to define and promote Translational Medicine among clinicians, basic Researchers, biotechnologists, politicians, ethicists, sociologists, investors and coordinate these efforts among different countries (5).

Different opinions have one single aim: the resolution of pathologies, thought the specific application for the patients, in particular for the research discovery of new drugs or vehicle of these. The interaction of several disciplines is required to translate knowledge from one type of research to another (e.g., to move a basic science discovery to the bedside). Collaboration among disciplines through multidisciplinary teams facilitates the appearance of novel concepts and approaches to discovery of important health issues. The development of new ideas are goals of translational research, and there are many possible models of training that can provide the academic path to these goals (4). Translational research is defined as "the process of applying ideas, insights, and discoveries generated through basic scientific examination to the treatment or prevention of human disease" (http://grants1.nih.gov/grants/guide/pa-files/PAR-02-138.html), sometimes abbreviated as "from bench to bedside" (http://www.nihroadmap nih.gov). Translational research should be regarded as a two-way road: Bench to Bedside and Bedside to Bench (6). Discovering better ways to ensure that patients receive the care they nee safely, compassionately, and when they need it is not easy and poses formidable methodological challenges. The core of definition, is translational that indicate the transfer, transduction of basic scientific results in new interesting application to improve the human health (7). The translation of the new knowledge, mechanisms, and techniques generated by advances in basic science research into new approaches for prevention, diagnosis, and treatment of disease is essential for improving health (8). This transfer is related not only to the capacity of scientist to identify the new area of research that have more interest for the human global health, but also the collaboration between different scientists that can help this transfer of knowledge. We didn't know at the time that there were any particular disease implications (9). Given the growing impact of scientific knowledge and discoveries on clinical practice, translational medicine was initially described as "the marriage between new discoveries in basic science and clinical practice" Basic research is performed without thought of practical ends.. It' is important to define the Basic research: It results in general knowledge and an understanding of nature and its laws. This general knowledge provides the means of answering a large number of important practical problems, though it may not give a complete specific answer to any one of them. The function of applied research is to provide such complete answers (10).

Basic science researchers excel at identifying unanswered questions in the field of medicine and play an integral role in increasing understanding of disease pathogenesis, therapeutic mechanisms, and preclinical development. However, the fundamental questions that basic scientists answer are not always directly relevant to any prospective form of treatment or clinical advance. Even though their work offers potential new medical insights, they do not endeavor to design and execute subsequent research to apply their basic science breakthroughs toward new medical technologies, diagnostics, or treatments for clinical application. In the contest of translational medicine we identify two area of interest: The clinical translational medicine. Clinical translational medicine (CTM) is an emerging area comprising multidisciplinary research from basic science to medical applications and entails a close collaboration among hospital, academia and industry (11). CTM is to bridge the divide between health informatics 'bench research' and the application of informatics in clinical and health care settings (12). The critical care community is beginning to adopt an increasingly translational approach to research, drug development and early-phase clinical trials (13). Translational research imply two areas of translation. The process of applying discoveries generated during research in the laboratory, and in preclinical studies, to the development of trials and studies in humans. The second area is about the research that aims to enhance the adoption of best practices in the community. Cost-effectiveness of prevention and treatment strategies is also an important component of translational science (14).

Goals
The establishment of guidelines for drug development of for the identification and validation of clinically relevant biomarkers.
Experimental non-human and non-clinical studies conducted with the intent of developing principles for discovery or new therapeutic strategies.
Clinical investigations which provide the biological fondation for the development of improved therapies.
Any clinical trial initieted in accordance with the above goals.
Basic science studies which define the biological effects of therapeutics in humans.

Table 1: Goals and areas defining translational research. Adapted from Clinical Science (2007) 112, 217–227 (Printed in Great Britain) doi:10.1042/CS20060108 Bruce H. LITTMAN, Linda DI MARIO, Mario PLEBANI and Francesco M. MARINCOLA.

Clinical and translational medicine should be defined and differentiated from the understanding of other "translational" concepts, including translational science, translational research, translational medicine, or clinical and translational science. In contrast to these definition , clinical and translational medicine is expected to concentrate on clinical application-oriented translational science and research to improve the accuracy, efficiency and efficacy of clinical diagnoses, therapies, and determination of prognoses for patients. The role of clinical and translational science and research is becoming more important than ever, as we attempt to meet the future needs of clinical and translational medicine, to form more global opinion leaders to bridge the gap between understanding basic science and human disease, and to define the content, regulation and policy of clinical and translational

6

medicine. The definition has facilitated cross-program efforts to identify core competencies, best practices, and meaningful outcomes that are relevant across the broad spectrum of training in clinical research.

Translational research fosters the multidirectional integration of basic research, patient-oriented research, and population-based research, with the long-term aim of improving the health of the public TR describes a continuum of research in which basic science discoveries are utilized to prevent or treat human disease. It is an iterative process wherein scientific discoveries are integrated into clinical applications and, conversely, clinical observations are used to generate research foci for basic science: the "bench to bedside and back to bench" approach.

The process of translational research can be summarized as follows: first, according to clinical practice, raising clinical problems and refining scientific questions; then, systematic and in-depth research, which integrates diverse disciplines, including epidemic study, basic research and drug discovery, is carried out; last, through research, the potentially effective strategies or methods for diagnosing, treating or preventing diseases are achieved and translated into clinical practice. Dr Marko-Varga emphasizes that the modern health care is undergoing a big revolution, where new therapies and novel technology advancements are having important improvement of patient care and managing costs. Certainly, the latest frontiers in micro and nano-technology which allows high resolution protein sequence separation as well as Mass Spectrometry imaging that can resolve drug deposition that are localized in tumor environments. One cornerstone within Health Care that has had great impact on cancer patients is the increasing number of personalized medicines being introduced into the market. The interest in personalized medicines actually results from understanding the molecular biology of diseases (15). Stephen I. Hsu (one of global leading scientists in translational medicine) emphasized that the topic of a "social mission" should be also important for clinical translational scientists, to think ahead about how to translate in a manner that will enable public health models for disease prevention or treatment in low-resource settings to be realistically and successfully implemented. High technology approaches can either produce expensive therapies with relatively small impact if the target population is small (gene therapy or stem cell & regenerative medicine for rare diseases, etc.), or it can produce affordable low-tech and self-administered therapies that are targeted towards addressing common diseases (e.g. pandemics such as obesity and its related complications such as type 2 diabetes, highly prevalent cancers prevented by novel low-cost screening and treatment) and are specifically developed to be effective and available to both the most wealthy and the most impoverished basic and translational science differ primarily in integration and practicality, respectively. The importance of basic science derives from its contribution to knowledge deeper within the tree of information and, consequently, its greater potential for integration with other events. In contrast, the importance of translational science lies in its practicality (16).

Brenner is one of many scientists challenging the idea that translational research is just about carrying results from bench to bedside, arguing that the importance of reversing that polarity has been overlooked (17). "We don't have to look for model organisms anymore because we are the model organism" he said. The question of how to define translational research remains actually unresolved and controversial. This is partly due to the different stakeholders attention for distinct aspects of this issue. For academia, translational research represents the potentiality to test novel ideas generated from basic analysis with the hope of turning them into useful clinical applications. For academic translational research also responds to the need of identifying novel scientific hypotheses important to human pathology through direct observation of humans and their diseases (6). For people more directly involved in clinical practice (physicians, clinical laboratory professionals and patients), translational research accelerates the capture of benefits of research, closing the gap between 'what we know and what we practice' (18). This means the transfer of diagnostic and therapeutic advances proven effective in large well-conducted trials to daily medical practice (19). About the commercial sector, translational research refers to a process that aims the development of known entities in the early phases and/or identifying ways to make decisions when the cost of product development is still contained. These opinions are not mutually exclusive and can overlap, although there are often differences between translational researchers with different goals and different definitions of success (20).

1.3 The 4 Steps of Translational Medicine
The iterative process where in scientific discoveries are integrated into clinical applications and, conversely, clinical observations are used to generate research foci for basic science: the "bench to bedside and back to bench" approach is described as follow. Initially, 2 phases in TR were described:

T1. basic science discoveries used to develop new treatments for disease ("bench to bedside"),(21)

T2. research aimed at improving utilization of proven therapies in clinical practice and community settings ("bedside to community").

More recently, this has been redefined to include 3 phases in TR, with the second phase being subdivided. Thus, in this new model T1 describes basic science to clinical science, T2 clinical science to clinical practice, and T3 is used to denote the translation of clinical practice to more widespread health improvements (22).

The translational paradigm could be sub-divided into four steps T1 research seeks to move a basic discovery into a candidate health application; T2 research assesses the value of T1 application for health practice leading to the development of evidence-based guidelines; T3 research attempts to move evidence based guidelines into health practice, through delivery, dissemination, and diffusion research; T4 research seeks to evaluate the "real world" health outcomes of a T1 application in practice (6, 23). Translational research encompasses the effective movement of new knowledge and discoveries into new approaches for prevention, diagnosis, and treatment of disease. Though the concept "translational research" is relatively new, the bedside-to-bench-to-bedside translational strategy is not original (24).

Translational medicine encompasses all the disciplines that intervene in moving scientific progress from the bench to the bedside and in conveying stimulating information from the bedside back to the bench (5).

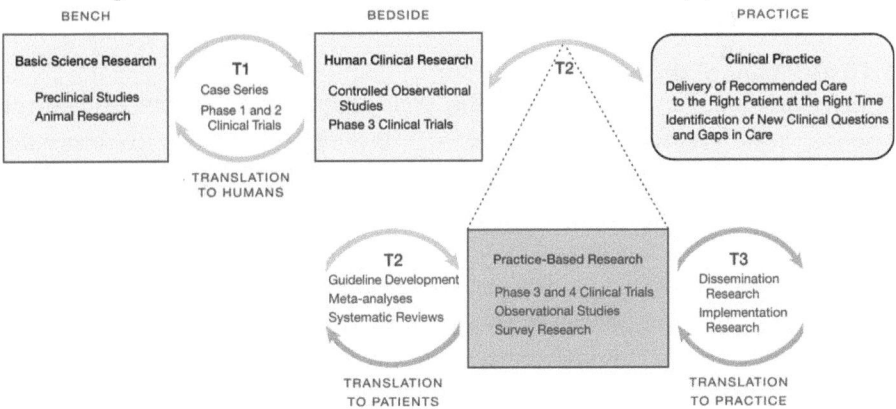

Figure 1: Adapted from John M. Westfall; James Mold; Lyle Fagnan JAMA. 2007;297(4):403-406 (doi: 10.1001/jama.297.4.403)

Within the T1 blockage sits the translational gap known as the "valley of death" (25-26).

The valley of death refers to the lack of funding and support for research that moves basic science discoveries into diagnostics, devices, and treatments in humans.

Awards were developed within the NIH to encourage collaboration between clinicians and basic scientists across institutes. But a more realistic approach would be to encourage opportunities to pursue Bedside to Bench research. Since our understanding of human disease is still limited and pre-clinical models have shown a discouraging propensity to fail when applied to humans. Translational research should be regarded as a two-way road: Bench to Bedside and Bedside to Bench. To promote translational research, it is required to set up translational research centers and cultivate a large number of talents who are engaged in translational research. Today, many translational research centers have been built up and numerous translational research programs have been carried out. These centers provide good hardware and the programs offer good human resources for translational research. Clinical and translational medicine integrates clinical research with modern methodologies in systems and computational biology, genomics, proteomics, metabolomics, pharmacomics, transcriptomics, and high-throughput image analysis. It should also foster the implementation of human tissue banking, and the development of bio-banks linked to high quality clinical database, for identification of clear phenotypes relevant to stratification of patients receiving standard or experimental therapies (27, 28).

1.4 The valley of death

The valley metaphor helps explain the impediments that prevent biomedical science from realizing its potential and the risks of failing to translate knowledge into public benefit. The impediments range from lack of technological innovation or "old style thinking" (26) to particular obstacles such as a lack of access to well characterized biological materials in biobanks (29) or insufficient training in translational science for the next generation of investigators (30). Biomedical research agencies are responsible for the first block in the progress of translational medicine. The really problems is that the clinical and basic scientists don't really communicate. As anyone attempting translational research will testify, basic scientists have few incentives to move outside their comfort zone. It means getting involved with complex regulatory and patent issues. There is the risk of career damage to boot, because it is not the sort of research that gets published by the top journals and spurs promotion. The pharmaceutical industry, which for many years was expected to carry discoveries across the divide, is now hard pushed to do so. The abyss left behind is sometimes labelled the 'valley of death' - and neither basic researchers, busy with discoveries, nor physicians, busy with patients, are keen to venture there. "The clinical and basic scientists don't really communicate," says Barbara Alving, director of the NIH's National Center for Research Resources in Bethesda (31). The basic biomedical research enterprise has now evolved its own dynamic, with promotions and grants based largely on the papers scientists have published in top journals, not on how much they have advanced medicine. And many clinicians who treat patients - and earn fees for doing so - have little time or inclination to keep up with an increasingly complex basic literature, let alone do research. This has diminished the movement of knowledge and hypotheses back and forth between bedside and bench. At the same time, genomics, proteomics and all its cousins are generating such a volume of potential drug targets and other discoveries that the pharmaceutical industry is having trouble digesting them (32).

Science and innovation have become too complex for any nostalgic return to the physician–scientist on their own as the motor of health research. Reinventing that culture is therefore the focus of the CTSCs, in the form of larger, multidisciplinary groups, including both basic scientists and clinicians, but also bioinformaticians, statisticians, engineers and industry experts. Zerhouni says he expects them to be breeding grounds for a new corps of researchers who will effectively stand on the bridge and help others across. Scientists at the centres will be evaluated with business techniques, such as milestones and the ability to work in multidisciplinary groups, rather than by their publications alone.

Molecular biology is a victim of its own success. Seemingly overnight, it has changed from a science of one gene, one protein, one molecule, one at a time, to all genes, all proteins, all molecules, all at once. Everything is now 'ome-sized. The generation and exploration of these data has become a massive, all-consuming discipline.

And yet the expected pay-off - the new therapies and diagnostics that will improve human health - has not kept pace. Researchers and funding agencies recognize this inequality and are working on a solution: translational research. The name encompasses the strategies by which the intellectual riches flooding from biomedical discovery can be converted into practical riches from which humanity can benefit. That team features experts in all aspects of clinical research, including medicine, pharmacology, toxicology, intellectual property, manufacturing, clinical-trial design and regulation. The basic researcher now has the back-up from those who can do the jobs for which he or she is unqualified. Translation is not a one-way progression in which research findings enter a production line and emerge at the end as drugs or diagnostics. The whole process is more fluid: experiments on human tissues and clinical trials can inspire fascinating new questions back at the bench that will, when answered, improve the human experiment in its next iteration (32). The application of science to the development of new medical technologies holds promise for eradicating diseases and personalizing health care. Effective translation from bench to bedside, however, requires that our major engines of biomedical research the academic medical centers work effectively with industry (33). This frustrating disconnect between making scientific discoveries and developing tangible medical applications emerged relatively recently (34, 25). Additionally, translational research performed by clinician-scientists often involves collaborations between government, industry, and private institutions, which makes it less likely that a project will be abandoned after an unsuccessful trial. However, many projects that fail to produce medically useful results succeed in generating new knowledge that may prove important. Further, the history of medical technology is replete with successful innovations that were initially considered insignificant, and the record of our best scientific c journals in accurately judging future benefits to human health is weak at best (35, 36) Many transformative technologies have been dropped by research teams and companies, only to be picked up later with eventual success (37). However, the resources needed are substantial, the costs high, and the failure rates daunting.

Questions for self-guided assessment of issues affecting the success of translational reseach projects	
Category	Evaluation questions
1. Is it worth the effort?	Does the new technology's intended use address a compelling health need? Is the scientific rationale strong, and does it sugget a possible medical benefit when compared with existing therapies?
2. Is there an adeguate potential commercial market?	Does the size and type of market indicate high likelihood of economic viability? Is the intellectual property protection solid? Is the technology likely to be cost-effective?
3. What can be inferred from human and animal data about likely safety and efficacy?	Is there a human genetic disorder that affects the tharapeutic target? If so, does the phenotype support the efficacy and/or safety of the agent? Are the animal models used to assess efficacy and safety convincingly representative of the humen disease?
4. Can the agent be delivered to its target at an adequate concentration?	Are the pharmacokinetics and pharmacodynamics acceptable for the intended use, based on direct assessment of the effects on the target molecule or measuringful functional assays?
5. Is there an industry partener that can develop the technology effectively and efficiently?	Is there an industry partner willing to make the development program a high priority? Will the industry partner ensure that the preclinical and clinical development groups exchange ideas throughout the development process? Is there an industry partner thet will refrain from excessive secrecy? Can the technology be manufactured easily and at a reasonable price?
6. Can a pivotal study be designed and completd?	Can a study be designed with a medically meaningful endpoint? Can the study be designed to reflect clinical equipoise and be attractive to both partecipants and their clinicians? Can a study be designed with sufficient statistical power to detect the endpoint?

Table 2: Adapted from John M. Westfall; James Mold; Lyle Fagnan JAMA. 2007;297(4):403-406 (doi: 10.1001/jama.297.4.403)

1.5 Personalized medicine : the principal tools of Translational Medicine

Translational medicine is thereby poised to identify the most effective science-based healthcare decision systems that align clinical care with individual patient and community needs. The emergence of clinical and translational science is represented from different issue as the paradigm to optimize medical as well as surgical products and services emanating from the intersection of discovery science and healthcare delivery, highlights the requirement for a unifying structure that bridges the knowledge creation and deployment, converting discoveries to human application, advancing that information into clinical practice, disseminating best clinical practices into communities, and modifying the behavior of populations to improve the wellness (38, 39). Individualized medicine is the principal goal of translational

13

medicine that aims to provide personalized solutions based on patient-specific molecular mechanisms of disease by transforming traditional healthcare practices that are applied to the population.

Tools of Translational Science in Medicine as backbone of an emerging science
New biomarker development e.g. imaging or serum parameters
Translational toxicology including more powerful biomarkers
Biomarker scoring systems to grade their predictive potency
Smart, early humen study design, including novel approaches e.g. microdosing and descriptive trials
Biostatistics development to cope with multiple read-out problems and small human sudies
Human genetics

Table 3: Adapted from Translational medicine: science or wishful thinking? Journal of Translational Medicine 2008, 6:31

To realize the personalized medicine is important identify new biomarkers The biomarkers are important to translational research because, ultimately, it may turn out to be the most effective way to reduce the cost of clinical experimentations while, most importantly, saving patients from ineffective and unnecessary treatments promptly redirecting them to treatments with higher likelihood of success. The Biomarker assay is associated to the drug, and the patient stratification. We are expecting that such drug products will prove to be more efficacious within the targeted disease process, but also free from unwanted side effects and toxicity. Biomarkers reflect biological effects induced by disease and/or a given drug and are the main tools to predict and describe its efficacy and safety (40, 41). Biomarkers include effects on serum parameters (e.g., the primary product of an enzyme which is inhibited by the drug), more general markers of disease severity (e.g. CRP and other markers in inflammatory processes (42)) but also imaging (e.g. plaque morphology in drugs affecting atherosclerosis, liver fat content as safety biomarker, or positron emission tomography (43, 44))or histology. These biomarkers are not clinical endpoints (such as death or myocardial infarction), which are the ultimate measures to demonstrate the efficacy of a drug, it is obvious that there are different categories of biomarkers (e.g. animal vs human) in achieving predictive power, and a classification seems desirable. They are ideally obtained first in animal disease models and then used in the equivalent human diseases to establish early confidence in efficacy and safety of a new drug or intervention. It is obvious that their predictive value can vary from almost useless (e.g. if one has to obtain serial brain slices, which will never become a human biomarker) to surrogate (e.g. LDL cholesterol, one of the few surrogates accepted by FDA), with most cases being somewhere in between. Obviously, such an objective, reproducible system should be superior to the common "gut feeling" approach towards judgment of biomarker utility, but this still needs to be proven. Early interaction between pre-clinical and clinical researcher is key in the development and validation of "good" biomarkers; the modern "-omic" techniques are very important in this context. Such human studies do not have direct regulatory implications, but should help a pharmaceutical company to develop the right targets as well as the right compounds. Disease understanding is another area where translational aspects have a tremendous impact and help to design or apply the right drugs for/to the right patient population. Translational medicine is charged with the determination of disease segments, using innovative bio- markers including genetics, which represent the optimal target populations for efficacious and safe drug applications. This is particularly important as cost effectiveness considerations are becoming increasingly competitive; they already represent reimbursement criteria and might even become a regulatory hurdle (45).

Translational medicine requires the full extent of patient data to be accessible so that questions spanning multiple data sources, such as those discussed above, can be asked and answered. For example, a physician in clinical practice would like to easily ask for the criteria for the diagnosis of a disease and the recommendations for personalized medicines.

1.6 Limits and opportunities of Translational Medicine

There are three major obstacles to effective translational medicine. The first is the challenge of translating basic science discoveries into clinical studies. The second hurdle is the translation of clinical studies into medical practice and health care policy (46).

A third obstacle to effective translational medicine is also philosophical. It is a fact that the available standard therapies for most common diseases are less efficacious than they are believed by the Public to be and significant funds are allocated to maintain. Finally, it may be a mistake to think that basic science, without observations from the clinic and without epidemiological findings of possible associations between different noxes and disease, it will efficiently produce the novel therapies that we are eager to test. If we as a body can coordinate efforts by advocacy groups, academia and industry to educate the public and the government of the need for translational medicine, novel and effective therapies could be the significant result (46).

There are some important aims about the translational medicine and in particular, build national clinical and translational research potential, Provide the adequate training and improving the career development of clinical and translational scientists, Enhance the collaborations, Improve the health of our communities and the nation; Advance T1 translational research.

Various M.D./M.B. Ph.D. programmes and master programmes, focusing on TR, are now also available and further training supported by dedicated fellowships are providing a clearer career pathway for both clinician-scientists and basic scientists. In the true translational spirit, both academia and industry should have the same goals, to improve patient care. Academics must become more business-driven; industry and academia can develop into much more similar and equipotent partners, and borders will become more permeable. Translational medicine seems to be an almost ideal vehicle to advance industry/academia collaborations, and complementary discovery/ development efforts in joint programs should be facilitated. The scientific process hopes to alleviate human misery and this ultimate goal could be facilitated by connecting basic scientists with the reality of human disease and making translational research more than an interesting concept (47).

Both in academia and industry, the wish to translate better has increased the awareness for interface problems; in academia, more clinical trials shall be performed as the tougher variant of medical research if compared with test tube research. Clinical trials require a lot more resources, paper work and endurance, and the rewards are still smaller in the public appreciation (papers, impact factors).

This challenge has been identified and a huge amount of money is now supplied to investigator driven trials in academia.

In industry, both preclinical and clinical studies have been performed routinely and professionally long before this call for translational activities emerged, now the major task is the intertwining and alignment of preclinical and clinical studies along the artificially straight drug discovery and development process. Here, it is more of an interface problem, than reflecting the lack of access to clinical trials. The main drawback of translational studies and related personalized medicine approaches in industry is the mandatory economical interest which is not in line with all sophistications of drug profiling leading to narrowed windows of opportunities. It seems that in some instances, such

16

translational efforts would have to come from parallel, independent, presumably academic IITs. In public science funding calls (e.g. EU Framework Program 7) or scientific meetings (e.g. Endocrine Society Meeting), "translational" seems to identify any proposal or topic which involves clinical material and non-established mechanistic approaches or early compound/medical device testing. Even epidemiology is coined as a translational medicine tool, if patient data are analyzed. Do those activities and interpretations of translational medicine live up to the expectations raised by the original motivation, namely to ultimately help patients? The threat to increased output is the fact that most activities under the umbrella "translational medicine" are pretentious and reflect phraseology, thus just wishful thinking.

Translational efforts are as old as medicine; all drugs on the market had a successful translational process in their history, and the wish to help patients by scientific tools has been around for as long as medical science exists. If the pressure exerted by lacking success just induces new terminology for old processes, it is simply not enough to warrant a major change. If success will not show, however, biomedical science could even become a major loser in the battle on investments into the future of mankind, given e.g. the environmental and energy supply threats.

It's very important to define the privacy patent. As translational research advances, it will drive a change in the very practice of medicine. Healthcare delivery is shifting from a retrospective approach, which is concerned with analysis of the root cause of failure ("what is your chief complaint?"), to a prospective posture based on risk assessment before the development of symptoms. This preventive approach has the obvious advantages of cost reduction and the improvement of patient prognosis (48). Translational research can identify relevant genetic or functional biomarkers predictive of genetic risk, capable of early detection and/or providing accurate prediction of response to treatment. Yet these studies are often limited by the need to protect individuals' privacy. It's very necessary an adequate training in Traslational medicine Translational researchers need special training in the complexity of new technologies.

Physicians must be sensitized to the complications of designing and conducting scientifically valid clinical trials. Scientists must be able to understand the ethical limitations of research when dealing with human beings. As these new frontiers in science emerge, a unified science curriculum that fully incorporates mathematics education and quantitative thinking has been proposed to prepare physician-scientists of the twenty-first century for the challenge of studying systems biology (49). An other important problem is represented by a lack of infrastructure and economic hurdles. The secret to success of translational research is teamwork, because the research endeavor requires that different skills be brought to bear on a unified goal (50).

One reasonable approach could be to link funding for translational research to spending on medical care. This would help to support the cost of institutionally approved clinical trials in cases where standard treatments do not offer a significantly greater chance for survival or improved quality of life. The goal of translational research is productive testing and validation of new therapeutic modalities or diagnostic and prognostic markers. The diseases that most impact US healthcare spending are chronic (51). The appropriateness of clinical or biological endpoints is often unclear (52) and multifactorial (53). Ideally, a biomarker informs clinical go-no go decisions, and serves to help optimize biological dose (54). Therefore, criteria are needed to identify markers that can be clinically useful, to assess the best methodology for clinical evaluation and to establish criteria to appraise the incremental value offered over standard prognostic factors (55). There is the complex issue of Identifying and validating surrogate markers for early go/no go decisions. The rate at which potential therapeutic targets are identified by modern biotechnology has increased the competition in industry for resources to test the efficacy of multiple drugs and mechanisms for the treatment of the same condition. Many new drug candidates target reduction in the progression of chronic diseases that require long and expensive clinical trials. For the realization of useful data, is important to plan a correct collection on patients sample. High-throughput technologies enable researchers to study human disease in its globality, accounting for genetic variability of individuals and the heterogeneity of their diseases. A major limitation, however, is the ability to link clinical information to high-quality sample collection. Although it is relatively easy to analyse genomic DNA (56), collection of material for functional genomic studies requires more planning of the optimal time frame for sample collection (before, during or after treatment) and is limited by the amount of material realistically obtainable from patients. Analysis of tissues affected by the disease process and targeted by therapy is difficult because it requires repeated biopsies. Yet, less invasive methods, such as serial fine needle aspirates, can be used to predict response (57) or to study mechanisms of action (58) using high-fidelity RNA-amplification methods

(59). Modern technology offers unprecedented opportunities in the clinical sciences (60). High-throughput technologies enable researchers to study human disease in its globality, accounting for genetic variability of individual patients and the epigenetic instability of their diseases. Extensive analysis of an individual polymorphism could complement information related to the disease process at the genetic, functional and post-translational level. Prospective collection of serum samples during therapy may help to identify patterns responsible for treatment toxicity and/or effectiveness. Application of standard practice for protein preservation using protease inhibitors and storage into appropriate aliquots are simple steps to ensure the usability of prospective collections. High-throughput technologies have revolutionized the ability to understand human pathology by computing thousands of factors simultaneously, limiting the inherent barriers to controlling variables in human disease. However, samples collected retrospectively are often unusable for analysis, as RNA degrades quickly after tissues or fluids are removed from the organism. The opportunity to take specific steps to preserve the *ex vivo* profile is often lost unless researchers know early that the sample in question would be useful for a particular in clinical study. It' s necessary to have an appropriate structure in which the academic organization research is performed and it is not suited to the efficient conduct of translational research, as different disciplines are separate from each other administratively, physically and culturally (61). The need for such interaction in translational research is better met by a 'project structure' that draws upon the talents of experts representing different specialties to create smoothly functioning creative teams (62). Translational research units should not be assembled according to similarity of scientific background, but around a mission-based goal. This congregation of talents can realize a solid structure in which each team member belongs to the same unit at the physical and administrative level and, most importantly, is rewarded according to the same review process. This should increase the cost effectiveness and running clinical trials from the primary conception, thought all principal steps.

1.7 Conclusions

There are many consideration about the translational medicine and its effect on clinical practice Translational medicine is a new point of vision of medicine and its applications. The explanation of translational medicine definition is indispensable at this time, in this era of progress of science. The importance to investigate the fundamental area of research and identify the potential application area is the most important objective to realize the really

19

application of years of knowledge in basic science. Translation medicine includes the individualized medicine that is the principal goal of translational medicine that aims to provide personalized solutions based on patients specific molecular mechanisms of disease by transforming traditional healthcare practices that are applied to the population and improve global wellness. This chapter analyzed the principal points of translational medicine and identify the way to go at to the future of medicine with translational basic information application for the obtainment of interesting results and more new applications. Through the knowledge of the 4 T, that represent the iterative process where scientific discoveries are integrated into clinical applications and, conversely, clinical observations are used to generate research foci for basic science, we could study new strategy. About the different point of 4T is important to consider the valley of death: this metaphor helps explain the impediments that prevent biomedical science from realizing its potential and the risks of failing to translate knowledge into public benefit.

Many progress have been made, but there are still now limits at the evolution of this concept of medicine. The really solution could be in the construction of the bridge between different professional figures that contribute at the progression of science and realize the effective strategy to resolve the data dispersion and absence of scientific communication.

It' s important promote the education at different level of competencies about the translation medicine definition and it's really application, that has effect on the progress of the society.

References

1. Zerhouni EA, "Translational and clinical science time for a new vision" New England Journal of Medicine 2005; 353(15):1621-3
2. Littman BH, Di Mario L, Plebani M, Marincola FM What's next in translational medicine?Clin Sci (Lond). 2007;112(4):217-27.
3. Anastasio A, Armenante A, Gimigliano A, Moscarino A, Panzera S, Romano R, Russo I, Scarpati G. To Be or Not To Be Translational Translational Medicine 2010; 85(3): 470–475.
4. Rubio DM, Schoenbaum EE, Lee LS, Schteingart DE, Marantz PR, Anderson KE, Platt LD, Baez A, Esposito K Defining Translational Research: Implications for Training. Acad Med. 2010;85(3):470-5.
5. Wang X, Wang E, Marincola FM.Translational Medicine is developing in China: A new venue for collaboration J Transl Med. 2011;2-4

6. Marincola FM. Translational Medicine: A two-way road.J Transl Med. 2003;1(1): 1479-5876
7. Woolf SH. The meaning of translational research and why it matters. JAMA. 2008 299(2):211-3.
8. Fontanarosa PB, DeAngelis CD. Basic science and translational research in JAMA. 2002;287(13):1728.
9. Rienzi, G., and A. Huang. 12 October 2009. Our newest Nobelist: Carol Greider. JHU Gazette, Johns Hopkins University,Baltimore.
10.Geraghty J. Adenomatous polyposis coli and translational medicine. Lancet 1996; 17;348(9025):422.
11.Bush, V., editor. Science: The Endless Frontier A Report to the President by Vannevar Bush, Director of the Office of Scientific Research and Development. Washington, DC: United States GovernmentPrinting Office; Jul1945 [Accessed November 13, 2009.]. Section 3 (The Importance of BasicResearch), Chapter 3 (Science and the PublicWelfare).
12.Qian M, Wu D, Wang E, Marincola FM, Wang W, Rhodes W, Liebman M, Bai C, Lam CW, Marko-Varga G, Fehniger TE, Andersson R, Wang X.Development and promotion in translational medicine: perspectives from 2012 sino-american symposium on clinical and translational medicine. Clin Transl Med. 2012; 1(1)-5.
13.Lehmann CU. et al. Translational research in medical informatics or from theory to practice. A call for an applied informatics journal. Methods Inf Med. 2008;47(1):1–3.
14.Schweikhart SA, Dembe AE. The applicability of Lean and Six Sigma techniques to clinical and translational research. J Investig Med. 2009 ; 57(7):748-55.
15.Xiangdong WangWang A new vision of definition, commentary, and understanding in clinical and translational medicine. Clinical and Translational Medicine 2012; 1:5
16.Fang FC, Casadevall A. Lost in translation--basic science in the era of translational research. Infect Immun. 2010 ;78(2):563-6.
17. Ledford H..Translational research: the full cycle. Nature. 2008;453:843-5.
18.Plebani M The changing scenario in laboratory medicine and the role of laboratory professionals in translational medicine.Clin Chim Acta. 2008;393(1):23-6.
19.Plebani M, Marincola FM. Research translation: a new frontier for clinical laboratories. Clin Chem Lab Med. 2006;44(11):1303-12
20.Michael R. Emmert-Buck Translational Research: From Biological Discovery to Public Benefit (or Not) Advances in Biology. Advances in Biology. Volume 2014.
21.Homer-Vanniasinkam S, Tsui J.The Continuing Challenges of Translational Research: Clinician-Scientists' Perspective Cardiol Res Pract,(2012) Volume 2012.

22.M. Westfall, J. Mold, and L. Fagnan, "Practice-based research—"Blue highways" on the NIH roadmap JAMA 2007;297(4):403-6
23.Khoury MJ, Gwinn M, Yoon PW, Dowling N, Moore CA, Bradley L.The continuum of translation research in genomic medicine: how can we accelerate the appropriate integration of human genome discoveries into health care and disease prevention? Genet Med. 2007 ;9(10):665-74.
24.Zhuqin Z., Houzao C & Depei L. Translational research: Lessons from past research, growing up nowadays, and development goal in future Life Sciences SCIENCE CHINA Life Sciences » 2011, 54 »(12): 1085-1088
25.Butler D. Translational research: crossing the valley of death. Nature. 2008;453(7197):840–842.
26.Coller BS, Califf RM. Traversing the Valley of Death: A Guide to Assessing Prospects for Translational Success. Sci Transl Med. 2009 9;1(10):
27.Wang X Role of clinical bioinformatics in the development of network based Biomarkers. J Clin Bioinforma 2011, 1(1):28.8.
28.Chen H, Song Z, Qian M, Bai C, Wang XD: Selection of disease-specific biomarkers by integrating inflammatory mediators with clinical informatics in AECOPD patients: a preliminary study. J Cell Mol Med 2011, 1582-4934.
29.European Commission: Biobanks for Europe - A Challenge for Governance. EUR 25302 Luxembourg: Publications Office of the European Union; 2012. (28)
30.Abedin Z, Biskup E, Silet K, Garbutt JM, Kroenke K, et al: Derivingcompetencies for mentors of clinical and translational scholars.Clin Transl Sci 2012, 5(3):273–280
31.Coller BS, Califf RM. Traversing the Valley of Death: A Guide to Assessing Prospects for Translational Success. 2009;1(10)
32.Collins FS: Reengineering translational science: the time is right. Sci TranslMed 2011, Sci Transl Med. 2011;3(90).
33.Califf. R. M. , Berglund L., Linking scientifi c discovery and better health for the nation: The maturation of clinical and translational research in the United States. Acad. Med., in press.34
34.Carmichael M, Begley S. Desperately seeking cures: How the road from promising scientific breakthrough to real-world remedy has become all but a dead end. Newsweek. 2010;155(22):38–43
35.Crowley F. Jr. Translation of basic research into useful treatments: How often does it occur? Am. J. Med. 2003;114, 503–505
36.Contopoulos-Ioannidis DG, Ntzani E, Ioannidis JP. Translation of highly promising basic science research into clinical applications. Am J Med. 2003 15;114(6):477-84.
37.Antman EM, Braunwald E. Am Heart J 2001 Dec;142(6):929-31.
38.Waldman SA, Terzic A. The roadmap to personalized medicine . Clin Transl Sci. 2008 1(2):93
39.Waldman SA, Terzic A: Clinical andtranslational science: from bench-bedside to global village. Clin. Transl. Sci. 2010 3(5), 254–257

40.Frank R, Hargreaves R   Clinical biomarkers in drug discovery and development. Nat Rev Drug Discov: 2003 ;566–580

41.Schonbeck U, Libby P Inflammation, immunity, and HMG-CoA reductase inhibitors: statins as anti-inflammatory agents? Circulation 2004;109(21 Suppl 1):II18–II26.

42.Stahl A, Wieder H, Piert M, Wester HJ, Senekowitsch-Schmidtke R, Schwaiger M Positron emission tomography as a tool for translational research in oncology. Mol Imaging Biol 2004; 6:214–224.

43.Luciano JS, Andersson B, Batchelor C, Bodenreider O, Clark T, Denney CK, Domarew C, Gambet T, Harland L, Jentzsch A, Kashyap V, Kos P, Kozlovsky J, Lebo T, Marshall SM, McCusker JP, McGuinness DL, Ogbuji C, Pichler E, Powers RL, Prud'hommeaux E, Samwald M, Schriml L, Tonellato PJ, Whetzel PL, Zhao J, Stephens S, Dumontier M. The Translational Medicine Ontology and Knowledge Base: driving personalized medicine by bridging the gap between bench and bedside. J Biomed Semantics. 2011 Suppl 2:S1

44.Mankoff S. P , Brander C, Ferrone S. and Marincola F. M Commentary Open Access Lost in Translation: Obstacles to Translational Medicine Journal of Translational Medicine 2004, 2:14 Journal of Translational Medicine 2004, 2:14

45.Wehling M. Translational medicine: can it really facilitate the transition of research "from bench to bedside"?Eur J Clin Pharmacol. 2006 ;62(2):91-5.

46.Jordan S Pober, Neuhauser C and Jeremy M.P. Obstacles facing translational research in academic medical centers The FASEB Journal vol. 15, 2303-2313

47.Abedin Z, Biskup E, Silet K, Garbutt JM, Kroenke K, Feldman MD, McGee R Jr, Fleming M, Pincus HA. Deriving competencies for mentors of clinical and translational scholars. Clin Transl Sci. 2012 ;5(3):273-80.

48.Bialek W., Botstein D. Introductory science and mathematics education for 21st-Century biologists. Science. 2004 ;6;303(5659):788-90.

49.Parks MR, Disis ML Conflicts of interest in translational research.J Transl Med. 2004:9;2(1):28

50.Snyderman R. AAP Presidential Address: The AAP and the transformation of medicine. J Clin Invest. 2004;114(8):1169-73.

51.Arteaga CL, Baselga J. Clinical trial design and end points for epidermal growth factor receptor-targeted therapies: implications for drug development and practice.Clin Cancer Res. 2003;9(5):1579-89.

52.Kluft C.Principles of use of surrogate markers and endpoints. Maturitas 2004;47(4):293-8

53.Martin JB, Kasper DLIn whose best interest? Breaching the academic-industrial wall. N Engl J Med. 2000 Nov 30;343(22):1646-9.

54.Conley BA, Taube SE.Prognostic and predictive markers in cancer. Dis Markers. 2004;20(2):35-43

55.Jin, P. and Wang, E. Polymorphism in clinical immunology. From HLA typing to immunogenetic profiling. J. Transl. Med. 2003; 1, 8.

56.Wang, E., Miller, L. D., Ohnmacht, G. A. et al. Prospective molecular profiling of subcutaneous melanoma metastases suggests classifiers of immune responsiveness. Cancer Res. 2002;62:3581–3586

57.Panelli, M. C., Wang, E., Phan, G. et al. Genetic profiling of peripheral mononuclear cells and melanoma metastases in response to systemic interleukin-2 administration. Genome Biol. 2002.

58.Wang, E. RNA amplification for successful gene profiling analysis. J. Transl. Med. 2005.

59.Rees, J. Complex disease and the new clinical sciences. Science 2002; 296, 698–700.

60.Horig, H., Marincola, E. and Marincola, F. M. Obstacles and opportunities in translational research. Nat. Med. 2005; 705–708

61.Mintzberg, H. Organizational design, fashion or fit? Harvard Business Rev. 1981; 103–116

62.Pope C, Mays N. Reaching the parts other methods cannot reach: an introduction to qualitative methods in health and health services research. BMJ. 1;311(6996):42-5.

CHAPTER II
Technological Transfer and translational medicine

2.1 Introduction

In this chapter:

2.1 Introduction
2.2 The definition and role of Technological Transfer in Medicine.
2.3 Conclusions

Translational medicine refers to the process by which the results of research done in the laboratory are directly used to develop new ways of patients treatment. It depends on the integration of the entire breadth of patient data with basic life science data to facilitate and evaluate drug development. Translational research encompasses the effective movement of new knowledge and discoveries into new approaches for prevention, e successful bench to bedside research, in particular for the valley of death resolution. In this context it' s very important the Industry and academy relation for the technological transfer realization.

2.2 The definition and role of Technological Transfer in Medicine

The key element to successful strategy in translational medicine application is the multidisciplinary approach to medicine problems (1). However real innovation is to have a continue connection between Academy and Industry to realize more practical discovery with real beneficial effects for the population. Governments have long encouraged university-industry collaboration, hoping to spur innovations that bring jobs, investment and life-enhancing products (2). Universities and academic health centers, that represent the major recipients of public investment in biomedical science, must translate new knowledge into applications that confer human benefit (3). In the University is possible to identify structures orientated to the knowledge diffusion, as incubators or technology parks. The success of business incubators and technology parks in the University settings is determined by how well a new technology is transferred from the laboratory to their startup firms. University technology transfer offices (UTTOs) function as "technology intermediaries" in fulfilling this role (4). For example, like most universities, the University of California requires faculty members and other researchers to disclose any invention that has commercial potential to one of its offices of technology transfer (OTTs), and to list funding sources for the project that led to it. Under these terms, an invention is anything that a researcher feels could be patented or is otherwise valuable as intellectual property: it might be a material, a method, or an animal or plant. The OTT then determines whether to pursue intellectual property protection on the university's behalf and negotiates contracts with potential licensees (5).

Another instrument to realize this transfer is represented by spin off organization. A *spin-off* is a new company that is formed (1) by individuals who were former employees of the parent organization, and (2) a core technology that is transferred from the parent organization. Spin-offs represent an important mechanism for technology transfer, as a spin-off is typically founded around a core technological innovation that was initially developed at the parent organization. It's represents a mechanism for creating jobs and new wealth (6). However, translating fundamental discoveries into practical applications takes many expensive, often highly regulated steps and these activities have generally not been a major focus of academic institutions. Since the Act's passage, virtually every university that is engaged in research has created a technology transfer office with the mission of helping the university commercialize their inventions. In the translational spirit, both academia and industry should have the same goals, to improve patient care. Academics must become more business-driven; industry and academia can develop into much more similar and equipotent partners, and borders will become more permeable. Translational medicine seems to be an almost ideal vehicle to advance industry/academia collaborations, and complementary discovery/development efforts in joint programs, should be facilitate the technology transfer process starts with "getting it" an inventor submitting an invention disclosure to the technology transfer office. The next stage, "know it," the technology transfer office reviews inventions submitted by faculty, staff and students to assess both the patentability and market potential of each one. For marketability or "use it," we look at the 'so what' factor. So what if we get a patent would anyone care or, more to the point, would anyone pay to license the patent from us? (1) It should be pointed out that not all inventors readily come forward with inventions; University inventions and discovery are playing an increasingly important role in economic development. Because patent prosecution can be expensive it is important to understand the market value of the invention before spending money to obtain an asset that may just sit on the shelf (1).

Technological transfer being a technology transfer professional allows you the opportunity to work at the interface of science and business and to help move discoveries forward for the public heath improvement (1).

2.3 Conclusions

To produce new useful discovery in basic science, it' very important to analyze the different area of medicine, and look to the potential investment that could create the bridge between the Industry and Academy and realize the applicative medicine. It' s important overcome the valley of death that refers to the lack of funding and support for research that moves basic science discoveries into diagnostics, devices, and treatments in humans. It' s necessary to fund research development that may not result in a drug or device that will be utilized in the clinic and conversely.

Moreover it' s necessary strengthen the link between laboratory researchers and industry.

References

1. SheftJ. Technology transfer and idea commercialization.Nat Biotechnol. 2008 26(6):711
2. President's Council of Advisors on Science and Technology University–Private Sector Research Partnerships in the Innovation Ecosystem (OSTP, 2008); available at http://go.nature.com/hilyum.
3. Mason Wright Freeman The Path from Bench to Bedside: Considerations before Starting the Journey J Investig Med. 2011 June ; 59(5): 746–751.
4. Morten Steffensena, Everett M. Rogersb, Kristen Speakmanc Spin-offs from research centers at a research university Journal of Business Venturing Volume 15, Issue 1, 2000, 93–111
5. Brian D. Wright , Kyriakos Drivas, Zhen Lei Stephen A. Merrill. Technology transfer: Industry-funded academic inventions boost innovation. Nature | Comment. 2014
6. Gideon D. Markman, Phillip H. Phanb, David B. Balkinc, Peter T. Gianiodisa. Entrepreneurship and university-based technology transfer Journal of Business Venturing . Volume 20, Issue 2, 2005, 241–263

CHAPTER III

Use of Animal Models in Translational Medicine

3.1 Introduction to Animal Models

The history of animal models goes back more than a millennium, when animals were used for experimental surgery. The first textbooks on anatomy were based on dissection on pigs and apes, not on human cadavers. Use of animal models is well known for some of the greatest discoveries in history. William Harvey's great work on circulation and Louis Pasteur's work in microbiology are few examples of use of animal model for great discoveries. Nowadays, the main use of animal models is for translational medicine and that role is considered the central point in the multidirectional paradigm of translational research. The advancement of medical field is greatly conditioned by the discoveries in pathobiology of human disease and drug development. Translational research is the process of transforming such discoveries into human application. Conventional experimentation in biomedical sciences had hitherto heavily relied on experimentation in vitro models such as cell culture and proteomic studies. Whereas in vitro studies offer distinct advantages for evaluating the effects on a cell system of a given factor in a biological system or a pathophysiological environment, the relevance of such findings to the whole organism is limited for many reasons. Whole animal studies are not only preferred for biomedical experimentation but rather essential for translational research. Developing animal models that simulate any given human disease is a crucial part of translational research and is the primary focus of this chapter.

3.2 Experimental studies in translational medicine

Scientific research implies the systematic and empirical investigation of hypotheses. In the biomedical sciences such systemic investigations may be classified as observational or experimental.

Observational studies are frequently (and most usefully) carried out when the variables influencing the outcomes of the phenomena under study either cannot be controlled directly or cannot be easily manipulated. These variables are, thus, carefully observed (occasionally over long periods of time) and an attempt is made to explain or determine the correlations between them. Examples include observing animals in their natural habitat and understanding how recent ecological changes impact on their survival.

Such observational studies also abound in clinical medicine and include descriptive case series, retrospective (case control) studies, prospective (cohort) studies and cross-sectional studies or surveys. These studies are particularly important where the conditions are rare and where it is important to understand the natural history of a particular condition (including the outcomes of currently accepted therapy). Investigations of these nature are also common in the basic biomedical sciences e.g. in molecular epidemiology and in comparative anatomy.

Experimental studies require intervention and attempts are made to directly control selected variables and to measure the effects of these variables on outcome. Such studies are necessary to establish cause and effect relationships in an unequivocal and rigorous manner. The results of experimental studies tend to be more robust compared to observational studies (although not necessarily more important) and many breakthroughs in the biomedical sciences are made possible only through experimental studies. Data arising from interventional studies also lend themselves easily to statistical analysis. The definitive experimental study in clinical medicine is the randomized controlled trial some of which can run into large numbers of patients. Clinical trials could of course also be carried out in non-randomized manners such as in sequential self controlled or cross over trial protocols. There are legislative requirements for most if not all new therapies (such as pharmaceutical and device related) to have undergone rigorous clinical trials before being accepted in mainstream medical practice and be considered standards of care. Experimental studies are similarly important in pre-clinical biomedical research. These studies may be carried out on in vitro biological systems such as isolated cells, cell culture systems, tissue slice preparations or isolated perfused organs. Experiments using in vitro systems are particularly useful in the early phases of studies where the screening of large number of potential therapeutic candidates may be necessary.

In vitro systems are, however, by definition, non physiological and have important limitations. Living creatures are biologically complex and this especially true in higher order animals including man. While data from experiments carried out in *in vitro* systems can establish mechanisms and define toxicities, *in vivo* biological systems using live animals (whole organisms) are necessary to study how such mechanisms behave under clinical or pathophysiological conditions.

Intact (whole) animal systems are, thus, extremely important for "proof of principle" research. It is frequently possible to have a clearer understanding of the efficacy, pathophysiological interactions and potential toxicities of novel therapies only with whole in vivo biological systems. Many *in vivo* interactions are complex and cannot be predicted from *in vitro* data. Such information is especially important when assessing the safety and efficacy of biologics. Biologics are therapeutics (drugs, vaccines, antibodies etc.) synthesized from living organisms. Biologics have made great advances in the last decade through advances in genetics and molecular biology especially recombinant DNA technology. Such therapies are increasingly developed and have contributed significantly to better outcomes in diseases e.g. in cancer therapy.

3.3 In Vitro experimentation and limitations.

Cell culture studies and tissue culture experiments are often performed to test a hypothesis or to examine the response of a cell or tissue preparation to a specific stimulus or inhibitory agent, often a humoral factor or a cytokine. Although such studies answer the question being posed, often with purity and precision, such observations have limited clinical significance. Often the cells used are derived from an established commercial cell line, which involves viral transfection and thus have altered cellular characteristics and the genetic composition. Cells derived from primary cell culture can circumvent this particular disadvantage but are relatively cumbersome to obtain and cannot be maintained past a few cell cycle passages. Often, studies performed in perfused isolated organs will provide more information than cell culture studies, but all the *in vitro* systems have the same major disadvantage: they lack the complex interactive physiology of the whole animal model. In particular, cell-cell cross talk and the paracrine and endocrine effects of the humoral systems in the whole animal facilitate and/or influence the responses of a specific cell or protein expression and activity. This is a major limitation in the interpretations of cellular responses in cell culture studies or tissue responses in the studies of isolated organ systems. Matarese et al (1) in their review showed that significant advancements have been achieved in understanding the dynamic changes that occur in vivo, both at the extracellular and intracellular levels. These dynamics can change at daily, circadian, weekly, or monthly intervals, yet they appear to follow defined temporal patterns. This greater understanding of cellular dynamics mandate that if *in vitro* approaches are to be used to emulate in vivo functions, the contemporary understanding of the continuously changing in vivo milieu must be adapted to in vitro approaches (Figure 1).

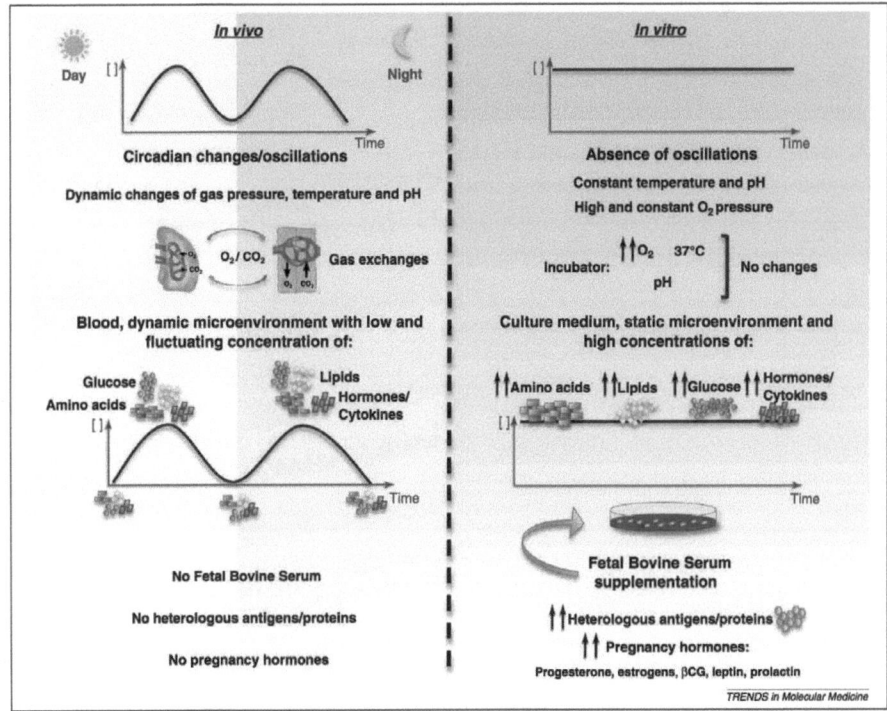

Figure 1: Schematic representation of the main differences between in vivo and in vitro systems. Typically, in vitro systems are static and not dynamic like in vivo systems. This phenomenon occurs for amino acids, glucose and lipid concentrations; hormones and cytokines; pH and temperature (1). These differences can dramatically affect experimental results that are often underestimated.

Numerous aspects and artifacts of *in vitro* culture systems represent a 'clear and present danger' to the insightful interpretation of results, as well as to an accurate determination of their relevance, and some of these issues are discussed in this interesting review. So they concluded that in vitro approaches have limitations that are often underestimated or not considered. The scientific community should be well aware of these aspects when interpreting data and should place a greater emphasis on developing in vitro new approaches that take into consideration the dynamic environmental and intracellular processes that are typical characteristics of normal physiology. Thus, whereas in vitro studies continue to contribute to understanding the pathophysiology of human disease processes and to drug development, whole animal models are crucial and pivotal for in translational research.

3.4 Animal Models for Translational Medicine

In biomedical research, an animal model is defined as "a living organism with an inherited, naturally acquired or induced pathological process that in one way or another closely resembles the same phenomenon in man" (2). The ultimate goal of experimental research using animal models is to solve problems in clinical practice and to develop new methods and approaches to the cure and alleviation of disease and disability (3).

Both invertebrate and vertebrate animals are used as models in biomedical research. *Invertebrate models* are very useful in the fields of neurobiology, genetics and development and notable examples of invertebrates use for such purposes include the *C. elegans* and *Drosophila.*

Vertebrate models are responsible for many advances in biology and medicine and are extremely important in translational research. This includes the use of both small animal models (e.g. mice, rats, rabbits) and large animal models (e.g. dogs, pigs, monkeys).

Broad areas of how vertebrate animal model are used in biomedical research include:

1. Pharmaceutical research including the development of biologics
2. Toxicology testing
3. Development and testing of new medical devices
4. Surgical research
   - the development of new surgical techniques e.g. techniques of gastrectomy, open heart surgery, coronary artery surgery, microsurgery, endoscopy and the use of arterial ligation in treating aneurysms (by the pioneer surgical scientist John Hunter).

- the development of new therapies e.g. organ and tissue transplantations, cardio- pulmonary resuscitation.

5. Pathophysiological research

Animal models were crucial to the understanding of basic and important pathophysiology processes such as shock and the body's response to trauma, regeneration and malignancy. In particular the development of the concept of the "milieur interieur" in physiology (by the pioneer physiologist Claude Bernard) and the concept renal dialysis all depended on the use of animal models.

The above is not exhaustive. The vast majority of animals used in biomedical research are in the fields of pharmaceutical research and toxicology testing.

When animal models are used for therapeutic testing, an established principle is to use the minimum number of animals necessary to arrive at scientifically robust data and to ensure the humane and proper care of animals so that the scientific data is reliable. Generally, two or more species (one rodent, one non-rodent) are tested because a drug may affect one species differently from another. Besides treatment efficacy, animal models are also used to determine how much of a drug is absorbed into the blood, how it is broken down chemically in the body, the toxicity of the drug and its breakdown products (metabolites), and how quickly the drug and its metabolites are excreted from the body.

3.4.1 What Makes a Good Animal Model?

Not all animal species are useful for the purposes of biomedical research and the limitations of the models selected as well as the methodology involved must always be kept in mind. Biomedical research is a very vast field and there are both general and specific uses for animal models. In the early years of biomedical research, animal models were mainly used for general research purposes i.e. to uncover broad pathophysiological phenomena and principles. The recent development and widespread use of transgenic animal models in biomedical research have made many animal models very specific to the nature of individual research projects.

While there are always exceptions, a good and useful animal model suitable for *general use* in a research facility should have the following characteristics (3-adapted from Isselhard, Kushe 1986):

1. The animal model should closely reproduce the disease or condition under study.

33

2. The animal model should be easily available to many researchers, that is, not a rare or exclusive animal. This allows validation and stimulates further investigations.
3. The animal model, in the case of a vertebrate model should be large enough for multiple biological sampling (tissue, blood etc).
4. The animal model should fit into available animal facilities of the average institution.
5. The animal model should be easily handled by most investigators.
6. The animal model should be available in multiple sub-species.
7. The animal model should survive long enough for results to be meaningful.
8. The animal model should be sufficiently robust for the purpose of the study.

Transgenic animal models, spontaneous animal models (see below) and highly specialized animal models such as non-human primates do not fit these traditional guidelines.

3.5 Consideration in the Selection of an Appropriate Animal Model
The researcher should consider using established models where possible or available (Table 1). The model must, however, be relevant to the aims of the study. The following serves as examples:
1. Relevance of species: For example, animals are suitable for studies on muscle contraction but data obtained from the whole body has little relevance to humans. In gastrointestinal tract and liver studies, herbivores have highly specialized gastrointestinal parts (e.g. for cellulose digestion) and associated metabolism, which has no counterparts in humans. Omnivores are, thus, most suitable e.g. pigs.
2. Numbers required: In studies where the outcomes between the control and study groups differ only in degree, large numbers of animals are required to achieve statistical significance. Mice and other small mammals are ideal.
3. Transplant and other immunological studies: Inbred or naturally immunosuppressed species may be required.

Examples of established general animal models	
Models	Species
Hemorragic shock	Rat, rabbit and pig
Stress Ulcers	Rat restrain model
Hypercholesterolaemia	Minipig
Sepsis Model	Rat, dog and pig
Primary Liver Cancel	Rat
Liver Regeneration	Rat and pig
Acute Pancreatitis	Dog and rat
Inflammatory Bowel Disease	Rabbit
Myocardiac Infarction	Baboons
Vascular Grafts	Dog, pig and sheep
Bone Fracture	Rabbit

Table 1

The animal model that is required to address the specific research question may, however, not have been previously developed or validated in some instances. The research effort must then begin by developing and validating a suitable model rather than using an established one. The development of a suitable model in this case becomes critical because it is essential that the model be reliable, reproducible and valid. The model must also be a reasonable representation of the actual situation and the limitations of the model must be identified. The validity of the results in experimental research depends on the qualities of the experimental model.

Occasionally, researchers may seek to use animal models that specifically mimic conditions of interest as opposed to using or developing general models. Such animal models may either spontaneously mimic these conditions or be induced to simulate those conditions.

- *Spontaneous animal models* are those models that have arisen through spontaneous mutations to mimic specific conditions. Notable examples of these are the Gunn rat (for hereditary hyperbilirubinemia) and the BB Wistar rats (for type I diabetes).

- *Induced animal models* can be created through surgical manipulations, chemical manipulation and genetic manipulations (including negative models). The surgically induced model is, in many ways, the classical biomedical research model and was used to understand brain plasticity (nonhuman primates), develop organ transplantation (dogs and pigs), discover the role of insulin in diabetes (dogs) and to develop card-pulmonary resuscitation (dogs).

Examples of chemically induced models include the chemical ablation of beta cells to create diabetes (rats, rabbits, pigs, monkeys) and the use of carbon tetrachloride to create cirrhosis (rats).

Transgenic animal models are important induced animal models. A transgenic animal is one that carries a foreign gene that has been deliberately inserted into its genome.

There are several varieties of animal models that have been used historically, and many of them continue to be used while recent technologies now facilitate development of many newer and refined animal models of human disease. Broadly speaking, there are 4 categories of animal models: (1) the inbred strains, which have been used extensively, (2) disease induction models, (3) xenograft animal models, and (4) genetically engineered models. Inbreeding has classically been used to obtain genetically homogeneous animals. Disease induction models are very commonly used to examine pathophysiology and drug development. Xenograft animals are used especially in cancer drug development. In general, to create a xenograft model, the tissue or an organ from one species is transplanted into another species. To make the animal more representative, it may be necessary also to inject human marrow cells into the mice to reconstitute the mice's immune system and "humanize" them so that their responses to a drug are more akin to those in a human tumor microenvironment. However, the development of genetically engineered models has made the most valuable contributions to this field. Genetically engineered models are developed by altering the genetic composition of an animal by mutating, deleting, or overexpressing a targeted gene.

3.5.1 Knockout Models

The knockout models are developed by knocking out one or several genes. These techniques have been so powerful and had such an impact on our understanding of human disease that the scientists who developed this approach won a Nobel prize. A detailed description of the techniques is beyond the scope of this manuscript, but the reader is referred to the cited references.

3.5.2 Transgenic Models

Transgenic animals are generated by inserting a desired gene into the model so the effects of such a gene can be studied on the physiology or pathophysiology of the animal. The genetic DNA can be inserted either into the fertilized egg or by injecting into embryonic stem cells, which are then cultured and introduced into the blastocyst. The transgenic modifications were originally performed predominantly in mice but are now routinely done in rats, primates, and other species.

3.5.3 Characteristics of an Ideal Model to Study Human Disease

Defining the characteristics of an animal model that is ideal for studying human disease is a major challenge. The most important requirement is the similarity of the disease pathogenesis in the animal model to the human disease process. However, verification of this implies detailed understanding of pathobiology in human disease, which creates a vicious circle for investigation (4). The situation is compounded by the fact that the molecular pathogenesis of many common human diseases such as hypertension and diabetes remains unclear until today. Dissimilarities in pathogenesis from human disease preclude suit- ability of an animal model for drug development for the human diseases in question. Furthermore, an ideal animal model should demonstrate the same biomarkers as in the human disease. This feature of biomarkers is important not only for monitoring disease progression but also for predicting drug toxicity.

3.6 Use of models to develop biomarkers of disease

Biomarkers are measurable parameters of biological processes and are very important tools in translational science. Some biomarkers reflect pathophysiology and may represent significant signaling pathways in the disease process. Thus, the presence of similar biomarkers in animal model and human disease indicates that pathogenic pathways are identical in both systems. The effects and effectiveness of a new drug can then be evaluated by the expected changes in the biomarkers further validating the animal models of a given human disease (5). Another important advantage in demonstrating useful biomarkers is earlier detection of adverse events in the course of development of a new drug (6). As discussed in the following sections, many animal models provide biomarkers for all the applications mentioned here.

3.7 Use of models for drug development and toxicity prediction

In the process of drug development, preclinical evaluation of the drug in animal models is not only very useful but quite essential before embarking on clinical studies (phase 1, phase 2, and phase 3 trials). This phase of the drug development in animals is necessary to demonstrate the anticipated therapeutic responses and to identify any adverse effect. However, a major problem is that there is a wide variability in development of toxic effects in different animal models, and many adverse effects observed in humans may not be seen in an animal model used for drug development (7). Thus, novel therapeutic agents, which are deemed safe and effective in animal models, may eventually turn out to be ineffective or even toxic in human studies. For example, aminoguanidine (Pimagedine), which is an inhibitor of advanced glycosylation end products is an illustrious example of this discrepancy.

Advanced glycosylation end products are very important in the pathogenesis of diabetic vascular complications and some non-diabetic conditions including aging. During the process of development of amino-guanidine, the preclinical studies in animals as well as clinical phase 1 and phase 2 studies established the safety and efficacy of the drug. However, in phase 3 studies, significant adverse events occurred in the final year of a 4-year study. Thus, un-expected occurrences of serious drug toxicity precluded the completion of phase 3 studies and sealed the fate of amino- guanidine as a potential drug.

In cases of certain other medications, the adverse events were not obvious even in the phase 3 clinical studies. In the post-market or phase 4 studies, toxic effects may be noticed, which were not detectable in the preclinical studies in the ani- mal models or in clinical phase 1, 2, and 3 studies. One such example is the experience with recombinant human erythropoietin. Epogen (recombinant human erythropoietin) was approved by the Food and Drug Administration rapidly after release of phase 3 data in view of its profound effectiveness to treat the anemia of chronic renal disease. However, occasional cases of Epogen resistance with pure red cell aplasia were reported in the first few years of its use in the dialysis population. In the following years, scores of reports involving hundreds of patients were reported or published. The flurry of reports related to these unanticipated adverse effect necessitated investigation into the chemical nature and manufacturing process of the compound and mechanisms mediating this adverse event.

Thus, an ideal animal model should be capable of demonstrating all the adverse effects that are observed in humans. This often requires the development of suitable biomarkers that can indicate the presence or development of an adverse event. On such biomarker is termed the kidney injury molecule 1 or KIM 1, which predicts the development of acute kidney injury equally well in both humans and animal models. The desirable characteristics of an optimal animal model are listed in Table 2.

Characteristics of an Ideal Animal Model of Human Disease	
1	Pathogenesis similar to human disease
2	Similarity in phenotypical and histological characteristics
3	Demonstrate similar biomarkers of disease
4	Reliable toxicity prediction
5	Similar response to proven therapies in human model

Table 2

3.8 Examples of Animal Models of Human Disease

Many animal species such as Drosophila and Caenorhabditis elegans have been used for replicating human diseases,(8) and they have yielded valuable information in understanding the pathophysiology of the disease and in drug development (9). For example, zebrafish is one of the species in which antiangiogenic drugs were developed (10,11) tested, and evaluated before human studies. Pigs and nonhuman primate are also used for these purposes and are particularly useful because of their sizes and proximity to human anatomy and physiology (12). However, rodent models remain the main species of animal models of human disease.

Several animal models currently exist for many human diseases such as hypertension, heart failure (13), atherosclerosis, stroke (14,15) and diabetes. Most of these models have at least some, often severe, limitations and deviations from the human dis- ease (16,17) and hence, there is an ongoing major effort to refine and improve them into ideal animal models. Invertebrates such as Drosophila have evolved as excellent models for studying patho- genic mechanisms and for drug testing in neurodegenerative dis- eases (18,19). Similarly, nonhuman primates have been used also as models of developmental psychopathology (20). Transgenic mice have been developed with selective knockouts of mitochondrial transcription factors to examine the mechanisms underlying neurodegenerative disorders (21-24). Furthermore, apolipoprotein E deficient and low density lipoprotein receptor deficient mice have been used successfully as models of atherosclerosis and drug development of the same (25).

3.8.1 Infections

Understandably, animal models are quite important in examining the pathogenic mechanisms of infectious disease and testing the safety and efficacy of antimicrobial agents. Accordingly, several models have been established in the recent decades to study various infections. For example, development of transgenic mice expressing hepatitis C viral proteins helped evaluate virus-host interactions and test new antiviral agents (26).

Diseases caused by Streptococcus pneumoniae are multiple and continue to be challenging. A recent review summarizes the techniques used in developing models of such diseases and how choosing appropriate animal models results in better understanding of these disorders (27). Another area where animal models such as mice, rabbits, and guinea pigs were used to study immunopathogenesis and efficacy of therapy is human tuberculosis (28). The major advances in pathogenesis of sepsis and demonstration of sepsis-induced tissue damage by novel biomarkers was described recently in the animal models of sepsis (29). Host responses to infection and factors that determine such responses have often been elucidated by optimal animal models as exemplified by certain mouse models of pneumonia (30).

3.8.2 Cancers

In the field of carcinogenesis and chemotherapy for cancer, the role of animal models need not be overemphasized. Human tumor xenografts have been useful in identifying tumor responsive histotypes and murine models have been extensively used in drug development and toxicology studies (31). Furthermore, the chemical basis of carcinogenesis was exemplified with N-methyl-N-nitrosourea (MNU)-induced gastric cancer in mice, which also provided more insights into pathogenesis (32). Because of greater similarity to humans in genetic aspects, immune system, and pathophysiology, nonhuman primates have been used in cancer research to the study the chemical and biological carcinogens. Such models are proving to be of great benefit, and the guidelines to optimally use them in cancer research continue to evolve (33). Additionally, animal models have been extensively used for determination of drug dosing using pharmacokinetics/pharmacodynamics data in cancer and non- cancerous conditions in humans (34).

3.8.3 Pulmonary Diseases

The understanding of several human pulmonary diseases and advances in therapy of such conditions has been significantly affected by development of suitable animal models. Such diseases include asthma (35) and other airway allergic disorders (36), idiopathic pulmonary fibrosis (37), pulmonary arterial hypertension (38), and chronic obstructive pulmonary disease (39). The characteristics of these animal models illustrate the importance of strategies to optimize such animal models to simulate human pulmonary diseases.

3.8.4 Liver and Gastrointestinal Diseases

In general, there has been a paucity of models of human hepatic and gastrointestinal disorders. However, in the last few years, spontaneous and induced models of primary biliary cirrhosis (40) as well as surgical, viral, and toxic models of acute hepatic failure (41) have been developed, which have aided in understanding not only the etiopathogenesis of these conditions but also transplant and other liver assist devices in the management of those conditions. Similarly, chemically induced models (42) and genetically engineered murine models (43) of inflammatory bowel disease have been used to study the pathogenesis and the efficacy of new therapeutic agents. Some nutritional issues, such as use of ketogenic diet in seizures (44), and biological mechanisms leading to complications of obesity have been evaluated in relevant animal models (45).

3.8.5 Psychiatric Diseases

Optimizing mouse models to evaluate the genetic basis and therapeutics of neurodegenerative diseases has been a challenging field (46-48) and has been well discussed in recent literature. Using animal models to evaluate predominantly subjective (49) and psychosomatic conditions is also equally complex and continuing to evolve.

3.8.6 Rheumatologic and Cutaneous Disorders

Mouse models of epidermolysis bullosa (50) and canine models of atopic dermatitis (51) have not only established the pathogenic theories but also have helped in rapid screening of new treatment options. A recent review summarized the usefulness of animal models of rheumatoid arthritis in identification of susceptible genes and examining the pathogenic pathways (52). Rat models of osteoarthritis have been used to evaluate new intra-articular drugs (53). The role of nitric oxide generated by endothelium through endothelial nitric oxide synthase in leading to endothelial dysfunction and contributing to vasculitis and atherosclerotic complications was established by transgenic mouse models (54). A vast array of findings has accumulated from animal studies to understand the basis of febrile seizures in infec- tive and other neurological condition (55).

3.8.7 Kidney Diseases

Many animal models have been used to investigate the genetic aspects of chronic kidney disease (56), pathophysiology, and drug development for various renal diseases including chronic kidney disease (57), podocytopathies (58), human immunodeficiency virus associated nephropathy (59), nephrogenic diabetes insipidus (60), polycystic kidney disease (61,62). Although these animal models may have contributed to understanding these disorders, there are several problems with these models that limit their usefulness. Notwithstanding such drawbacks, in many renal disorders, animal models have provided great insights. One example is diabetic nephropathy.

3.8.8 Animal Models of Diabetic Nephropathy

The following section focuses on animal models that are used to study the pathogenesis of diabetic nephropathy as an example of a common human disease and also because that has been the focus of our laboratory. These models may simulate nephropathy in type 1 and type 2 diabetes (63), and these may be derived from rodents, (mice and rats) as well as pigs and non-human primates. As in most conditions, rodents are the most extensively used species to examine this disease, especially after the advent of the transgenic and knockout technology. Type 1 diabetes is often induced by streptozotocin injection into rats (64) and mice, whereas type 2 is often due to genetic manipulations (65). Driven by the need to develop models to simulate diabetic complications, National Institute of Diabetes and Digestive and Kidney Diseases/National Institutes of Health funded a major initiative termed Animal Models of Diabetes Complication Consortium (AMDCC). Several studies funded by the AMDCC initiative were focused on transgenic and knockout mouse models and help us to further our understanding of the pathophysiology and pathogenesis of diabetic nephropathy. A detailed review of these models is beyond the scope of this manuscript. Models like db/db mouse and eNOS knockout helped us in the standing the significance of several mediators of pathogenesis, but none of the models could replicate the human diabetic nephropathy entirely.

3.8.9 ZSF Rats

After examining several popular models of diabetic nephropathy In our laboratory, we characterized the renal disease in ZSF rat and a newer rodent model of obesity and diabetes. ZSF rats were developed in Indiana University by crossbreeding rat strains with 2 separate leptin receptor mutation, Zucker di- abetic fatty rat and lean male spontaneously hypertensive heart failureYprone rat, derived from the obese spontaneously hyper- tensive rat. Phenotypically, they are normal until the eighth week when they start developing hypertension and spontaneous hyperglycemia, obesity, and hyperlipidemia, particularly hypertriglyceridemia. The renal manifestations develop pari passu with the other features; however, they become full blown after the 12th week (66). Initial hyperfiltration with subsequent decreasing renal function, increasing proteinuria, and progressive systemic hypertension accompanied by histological pictures of thickened glomerular basement membrane, mesangial expansion, arteriolar sclerosis, and diffuse glomerulosclerosis completes the renal manifestations in this model. Furthermore, many therapies shown to be effective in humans in slowing the progression of diabetic nephropathy such as glycemic and blood pressure control and inhibitors of renin angiotensin system are also very effective therapies in ZSF rats. Thus, ZSF rats represent an excellent model to study the pathogenesis and potential new therapies in diabetic nephropathy.

3.9 Translatability Score

In view of the myriads of problems encountered during preclinical and clinical phases of drug development, a scoring system was recently developed to minimize the challenges due to attrition of projects in tertiary stages and to enhance the translat- ability of potential drugs (67). A scoring system takes into account several factors including the preclinical (68) and clinical studies, biomarker validation, genetics (69), and pharmacogenomics (70) and scored to 1 to 5 times a weighted factor (Table 3). Such scoring system may be used at the stage of animal model selection.

Determinants of Translatability	
1	Initial evidence: invitro and in vivo experimental data
2	Human evidence: Genetics aspects, clinical trials
3	Biomarkers: Grading and development for efficacy and toxicity
4	Proof of concept testing
5	Pharmacogenetic data
6	Clinical aspects (unmet clinical needs, competitors)

Table 3

3.10 Limitations of Animal Models in Translational Medicine

Similar to human clinical studies, use of animal models for translational research with the goal of translation of bench research to clinic has few limitations. Involving young and healthy animals for research always carries a risk of selection bias. Natural dissimilarities between physiological and pathological system of various animal models and humans is one of the challenges of translation of bench research to clinical practice. Various remedies and approaches are underway to circumvent these differences. This includes work at the genetic, molecular, cellular, and clinical scale to understand the link between these elements within animals and humans. The ultimate goal of translating data between species via interdisciplinary approach will require techniques and expertise from mouse genetics, stem cell science, clinical research, comparative genomics, pathology, and medicine.

3.11 Conclusion

In the present era, animal modeling is considered the backbone of understanding various disease pathophysiologies and provides enormous opportunities for novel, effective therapy for a wide spectrum of presently untreatable disease and injuries. Recent advances in molecular technology are leading to the development of superior animal models and providing unprecedented opportunities to test both gene and pharmacological therapies prior to clinical trials in humans.

In conclusion, animal models of human disease are crucial for translational research studies and particularly those involving the development of novel therapeutic agents. Included in such animal studies are biomarker development and toxicity prediction. Many drugs often fail in phase 2 and phase 3 human studies owing to lack of accurate toxicity prediction, which in turn is often due to the lack of an ideal animal model for the disease state for

44

which the drug is being studied. To avoid enormous costs involved in drug development for various human diseases, some investigators have proposed a scoring model for translatability. However, the use of these scores still remains to be validated. The salient criteria that need to be considered while selecting the suitable and right animal model for translational studies were discussed in this review. Although the existing models represent powerful tools for translational research, several problems with them continue to challenge us. Thus, even with recent technological advances in animal model design, this area remains a fertile field for ongoing research and development.

References

1. Matarese G, La Cava A, Horvath TL. In vivo veritas, in vitro artificia. Trends Mol Med. 2012 Aug;18(8):439-42.
2. Wessler S. Introduction: What is a model?, pp. xi-xvi. IN: Animal Models of Thrombosis and Hemorrhagic Diseases. NIH, Bethesda, 1976.
3. Shimahara Y, Isselhard W. Evaluation of a short-time, oxygen carrier-free perfusion model in rat liver: mitochondrial energy metabolism and insulin effect. J Surg Res 1986 Jan;40(1):69-76
4. Persidsky Y, Fox H. Battle of animal models. J Neuroimmune Pharmacol. 2007;2:171-177.
5. Niederberger E, Geisslinger G. The IKK-NF-kappaB pathway: a source for novel molecular drug targets in pain therapy? FASEB J 2008;22:3432-3442.
6. Noiri E, Doi K, Negishi K, et al. Urinary fatty acid-binding protein 1: an early predictive biomarker of kidney injury. Am J Physiol Renal Physiol. 2009;296:669-679.
7. Storer RD, Sistare FD, Reddy MV, et al. An industry perspective on the utility of short-term carcinogenicity testing in transgenic mice in pharmaceutical development. Toxicol Pathol. 2010;38:51-61.
8. Wolozin B, Gabel C, Ferree A, et al. Watching worms whither: modeling neurodegeneration in C. elegans. Prog Mol Biol Transl Sci. 2011;100:499-514.
9. Iijima-Ando K, Iijima K. Transgenic Drosophila models of Alzheimer's disease and tauopathies. Brain Struct Funct. 2010;214:245-262.

10. Bell AJ, McBride SM, Dockendorff TC. Flies as the ointment: Drosophila modeling to enhance drug discovery. Fly (Austin). 2009; 3:39-49.

11. Park J, Kim Y, Chung J. Mitochondrial dysfunction and Parkinson's disease genes: insights from Drosophila. Dis Model Mech. 2009; 2:336-340.

12. Lunney JK. Advances in swine biomedical model genomics. Int J Biol Sci. 2007;3:179-184.

13. Zaragoza C, Gomez-Guerrero C, Martin-Ventura JL, et al. Animal models of cardiovascular diseases. J Biomed Biotechnol. 2011; 2011:497841.

14. Bailey EL, McCulloch J, Sudlow C, et al. Potential animal models of lacunar stroke: a systematic review. Stroke. 2009;40:451-458.

15. Daugherty A, Poduri A, Chen X, et al. Genetic variants of the renin angiotensin system: effects on atherosclerosis in experimental models and humans. Curr Atheroscler Rep. 2010;12:167-173.

16. Lynch WJ, Nicholson KL, Dance ME, et al. Animal models of substance abuse and addiction: implications for science, animal welfare, and society. Comp Med. 2010;60:177-188.

17. Lynch VJ. Use with caution: developmental systems divergence and potential pitfalls of animal models. Yale J Biol Med. 2009;82:53-66.

18. Lu B, Vogel H. Drosophila models of neurodegenerative diseases. Annu Rev Pathol. 2009;4:315-342.

19. Torres-Aleman I. Mouse models of Alzheimer's dementia: current concepts and new trends. Endocrinology. 2008;149:5952-5957.

20. Nelson EE, Winslow JT. Non-human primates: model animals for developmental psychopathology. Neuropsychopharmacology. 2009;34:90-105.

21. Harvey BK, Wang Y, Hoffer BJ. Transgenic rodent models of Parkinson's disease. Acta Neurochir Suppl. 2008;101:89-92.

22. Harvey BK, Richie CT, Hoffer BJ, et al. Transgenic animal models of neurodegeneration based on human genetic studies. J Neural Transm. 2011;118:27-45.

23. Elder GA, Gama Sosa MA, De Gasperi R. Transgenic mouse models of Alzheimer's disease. Mt Sinai J Med. 2010;77:69-81.

24. Gagliardi C, Bunnell BA. Large animal models of neurological disorders for gene therapy. ILAR J. 2009;50:128-143.

25. Zadelaar S, Kleemann R, Verschuren L, et al. Mouse models for atherosclerosis and pharmaceutical modifiers. Arterioscler Thromb Vasc Biol. 2007;27:1706-1721.
26. Barth H, Robinet E, Liang TJ, et al. Mouse models for the study of HCV infection and virus-host interactions. J Hepatol. 2008;49:134-142.
27. Chiavolini D, Pozzi G, Ricci S. Animal models of Streptococcus pneumoniae disease. Clin Microbiol Rev. 2008;21:666-685.
28. Dharmadhikari AS, Nardell EA. What animal models teach humans about tuberculosis. Am J Respir Cell Mol Biol. 2008;39:503-508.
29. Doi K, Leelahavanichkul A, Yuen PS, et al. Animal models of sepsis and sepsis-induced kidney injury. J Clin Invest. 2009;119:2868-2878.
30. Mizgerd JP, Skerrett SJ. Animal models of human pneumonia. Am J Physiol Lung Cell Mol Physiol. 2008;294:387-398.
31. Talmadge JE, Singh RK, Fidler IJ, et al. Murine models to evaluate novel and conventional therapeutic strategies for cancer. Am J Pathol. 2007;170:793-804.
32. Tsukamoto T, Mizoshita T, Tatematsu M. Animal models of stomach carcinogenesis. Toxicol Pathol. 2007;35:636-648.
33. Xia HJ, Chen CS. Progress of non-human primate animal models of cancers. Dongwuxue Yanjiu. 2011;32:70-80.
34. Mager DE, Woo S, Jusko WJ. Scaling pharmacodynamics from in vitro and preclinical animal studies to humans. Drug Metab Pharmacokinet. 2009;24:16-24.
35. Bates JH, Rincon M, Irvin CG. Animal models of asthma. Am J Physiol Lung Cell Mol Physiol. 2009;297:401-410.
36. Maes T, Provoost S, Lanckacker EA, et al. Mouse models to unravel the role of inhaled pollutants on allergic sensitization and airway inflammation. Respir Res. 2010;11:7.
37. Moore BB, Hogaboam CM. Murine models of pulmonary fibrosis. Am J Physiol Lung Cell Mol Physiol. 2008;294:152-160.
38. Stenmark KR, Meyrick B, Galie N, et al. Animal models of pulmonary arterial hypertension: the hope for etiological discovery and pharmacological cure. Am J Physiol Lung Cell Mol Physiol. 2009; 297:1013-1032.
39. Wright JL, Cosio M, Churg A. Animal models of chronic obstructive pulmonary disease. Am J Physiol Lung Cell Mol Physiol. 2008; 295:1-15.

40. Chuang YH, Ridgway WM, Ueno Y, et al. Animal models of primary biliary cirrhosis. Clin Liver Dis. 2008;12:333-347; ix.
41. Tunon MJ, Alvarez M, Culebras JM, et al. An overview of animal models for investigating the pathogenesis and therapeutic strategies in acute hepatic failure. World J Gastroenterol. 2009;15:3086-3098.
42. Kawada M, Arihiro A, Mizoguchi E. Insights from advances in research of chemically induced experimental models of human inflammatory bowel disease. World J Gastroenterol. 2007;13:5581-5593.
43. Mizoguchi A, Mizoguchi E. Animal models of IBD: linkage to human disease. Curr Opin Pharmacol. 2010;10:578-587.
44. Holmes GL. What constitutes a relevant animal model of the ketogenic diet? Epilepsia. 2008;49(suppl 8):57-60.
45. Kanasaki K, Koya D. Biology of obesity: lessons from animal models of obesity. J Biomed Biotechnol. 2011;2011:197636.
46. Chadman KK, Yang M, Crawley JN. Criteria for validating mouse models of psychiatric diseases. Am J Med Genet B Neuropsychiatr Genet. 2009;150B:1-11.
47. Gupta UD, Katoch VM. Animal models of tuberculosis for vaccine development. Indian J Med Res. 2009;129:11-18.
48. Patel V, Chowdhury R, Igarashi P. Advances in the pathogenesis and treatment of polycystic kidney disease. Curr Opin Nephrol Hypertens. 2009;18:99-106.
49. Pacharinsak C, Beitz A. Animal models of cancer pain. Comp Med. 2008;58:220-233.
50. Sitaru C. Experimental models of epidermolysis bullosa acquisita. Exp Dermatol. 2007;16:520-531.
51. Marsella R, Girolomoni G. Canine models of atopic dermatitis: a useful tool with untapped potential. J Invest Dermatol. 2009; 129:2351-2357.
52. Ahlqvist E, Hultqvist M, Holmdahl R. The value of animal models in predicting genetic susceptibility to complex diseases such as rheumatoid arthritis. Arthritis Res Ther. 2009;11:226.
53. Allen KD, Adams SB, Setton LA. Evaluating intra-articular drug delivery for the treatment of osteoarthritis in a rat model. Tissue Eng Part B Rev. 2010;16:81-92.
54. Atochin DN, Huang PL. Endothelial nitric oxide synthase transgenic models of endothelial dysfunction. Pflugers Arch. 2010;460:965-974.

55. Koyama R, Matsuki N. Novel etiological and therapeutic strategies for neurodiseases: mechanisms and consequences of febrile seizures: lessons from animal models. J Pharmacol Sci. 2010;113:14-22.
56. Garrett MR, Pezzolesi MG, Korstanje R. Integrating human and rodent data to identify the genetic factors involved in chronic kidney disease. J Am Soc Nephrol. 2010;21:398-405l.
57. Ichihara A, Sakoda M, Kurauchi-Mito A, et al. Drug discovery for overcoming chronic kidney disease (CKD): new therapy for CKD by a (pro)renin-receptor-blocking decoy peptide. J Pharmacol Sci. 2009;109:20-23.
58. Pippin JW, Brinkkoetter PT, Cormack-Aboud FC, et al. Inducible rodent models of acquired podocyte diseases. Am J Physiol Renal Physiol. 2009;296:F213-229.
59. Rosenstiel P, Gharavi A, D'Agati V, et al. Transgenic and infectious animal models of HIV-associated nephropathy. J Am Soc Nephrol. 2009;20:2296-2304.
60. Verkman AS. Dissecting the roles of aquaporins in renal pathophysiology using transgenic mice. Semin Nephrol. 2008;28: 217-226.
61. Belibi FA, Edelstein CL. Novel targets for the treatment of autosomal dominant polycystic kidney disease. Expert Opin Investig Drugs. 2010;19:315-328.
62. Harris PC. 2008 Homer W. Smith Award: insights into the pathogenesis of polycystic kidney disease from gene discovery. J Am Soc Nephrol. 2009;20:1188-1198.
63. Thayer TC, Wilson SB, Mathews CE. Use of nonobese diabetic mice to understand human type 1 diabetes. Endocrinol Metab Clin North Am. 2010;39:541-561.
64. Buschard K. What causes type 1 diabetes? Lessons from animal models. APMIS Suppl. 2011;132:1-19.
65. Brosius FC 3rd, Alpers CE, Bottinger EP, et al. Animal models of diabetic complications, C: mouse models of diabetic nephropathy. J Am Soc Nephrol. 2009;20:2503-2512.
66. Prabhakar S, Starnes J, Shi S, et al. Diabetic nephropathy is associated with oxidative stress and decreased renal nitric oxide production. J Am Soc Nephrol. 2007;18:2945-2952.
67. Wehling M. Assessing the translatability of drug projects: what needs to be scored to predict success? Nat Rev Drug Discov. 2009;8:541-546.

68. Deb KD, Sarda K. Human embryonic stem cells: preclinical perspectives. J Transl Med. 2008;6:7.
69. Dahme T, Katus HA, Rottbauer W. Fishing for the genetic basis of cardiovascular disease. Dis Model Mech. 2009;2:18-22.
70. Lee NH. Physiogenomic strategies and resources to associate genes with rat models of heart, lung and blood disorders. Exp Physiol. 2007;92:992-1002.

Chapter IV
New technologies in Translational Medicine

4.1 Introduction to translational research

In the last decade, new technologies have more frequently multidisciplinary approaches but the most important difference from use of different knowledge to translational medicine is the therapeutic index in human and/or the increase in human drug targets.

In this context, the translational research is probably the most important activity of translational medicine because integrate pharmacology tools, clinical methods, innovative technologies and studies of design to improve the progress of the translational medicine. It provides the knowledge necessary to draw important conclusions from clinical testing regarding disease and the viability of novel drug mechanisms. Different stakeholders give different definitions of translational research; we can say that translational research conduct experimental non-human and non-clinical studies with the intent of developing principles for new therapeutic strategies, but also for the development of improved therapies (1).

This approach has not few difficulties; one of them is the extensive investments placed for the private but also for the public sector. Besides, translational research encompasses a complexity of scientific, financial, ethical, regulatory, legislative and practical hurdles that need to be addressed at several levels to make the process efficient (1, 2).

Some of the obstacles faced by translational research include the fragmented infrastructure, lack of congressional and public support and more than ever high costs. Resistance also comes from those more familiar with traditional clinical research methods. In biomedical research, as it supports predictions about probable drug activities across species and is especially important when compounds with unprecedented drug targets are brought to humans for the first time but we think that translational research should be seen as enabled by ongoing efforts in basic and clinical research and not competing with them (1-3).

Several have resisted the idea of supporting translational research because of the fear that it may re-direct funds from other biomedical disciplines and of its high costs. Novel technologies based on high-throughput genomic and proteomic assays allow an effective search for novel hypotheses relevant to human disease by taking a global view of the phenomena associated with a disease and its response to therapy. In this way, it is possible use for translational research a new approach where the experimental heterogeneity associated with the uncontrollable genetic variability of humans and their diseases in its own favor, sorting common patterns necessary for the occurrence of a biological phenomenon from irrelevant ones. Development and diffusion can then be taken back to the bench for testing according to standard experimental models So, new technologies are very important for the translational research, especially if these technologies start yet from a multidisciplinary approaches, in these cases it is easier to improve them for the translational medicine (1-4). Here, there are some of them:

Nanotechnology is a multidisciplinary science that covers vast and diverse areas of devices derived from engineering, physics, chemistry, and biology. Nanotechnology was born with the use of nanoscale structures and materials as nanoparticles, nanowires, nanofibers, nanotubes. In particular nano-biotechnology is the application of nanotechnology in biological fields, for many biological applications (biosensing, biological separation, molecular imaging, anticancer therapy) using rapid advances of Nanotechnology in science and technology, creating new opportunities for advances in the fields of medicine, electronics, foods, and the environment (5). In medicine field and in diagnosis, detection of diseased cells would be faster, possibly at the point of a single sick cell, while allowing diseased cells to be cured at once before they spread into and affect other parts of the body. In addition, individuals suffering from major traumatic injuries or impaired organ functions could benefit from the use of nanomedicine (6).

Proteomic has a very important role in creating a predictive, preventative, and personalized approach to medicine. In this context the translational medicine uses the proteomic as a tool, because through the study of biological systems on a global levels is easier knock out the walls of several branch of science (7). This growing discipline integrates large and disparate data types, and deals with the infrastructural changes necessary to carry out systems biology bringing forth a new set of challenges for advancing science and technology (8-10).

New important technologies are represented by protein microarrays, a versatile platform for characterization of hundreds of thousands of proteins in a parallel and high-throughput manner. It is a new tool, which overcomes the limitation of DNA microarrays. In this case, all applications, viewed for proteomic are also used in protein microarrays for functional and structural applications. In addition, tissue or cell lysates can also be directly spotted on a slide to form the so-called "reverse-phase" protein microarray On the basis of its application, protein microarrays fall into two major classes: analytical and functional. In the last decade, applications of functional in particular it has flourished in studying protein function and construction of networks and pathways and so both for basic and for clinical research in diagnostic fields (11, 12).

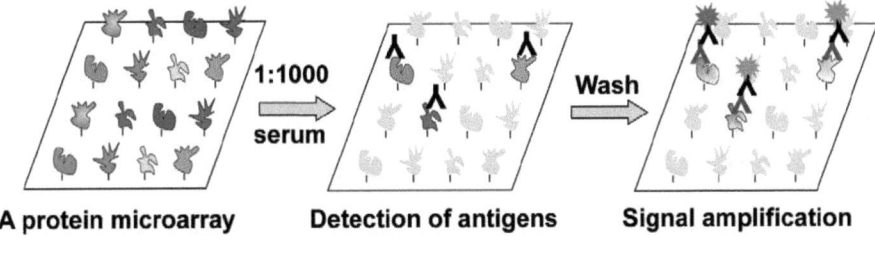

A protein microarray   **Detection of antigens**   **Signal amplification**

Labeled anti-human IgG, IgM, or IgA antibodies

Figure 1. Principle of serum profiling assays performed on a functional protein microarray. A functional protein microarray, composed of hundreds of thousands of individually purified proteins, is first blocked with BSA in PBS buffer. Then, a diluted serum sample is incubated on the microarray typically at RT for 1 hr. After extensive washes, bound antibodies (e.g., human IgG, IgA, or IgM) can be detected with anti-human immunoglobulin antibodies, followed by a signal amplification step with fluorescently labeled secondary antibodies. Detection of immunoglobulin isotypes can be multiplexed with different fluorophores as illustrated (12).

Regenerative medicine is a rapidly evolving multidisciplinary, translational research enterprise whose explicit purpose is to advance technologies for the repair and replacement of damaged cells, tissues, and organs. We can say about "regenerative pharmacology" describe the enormous possibilities that could occur at the interface between pharmacology, regenerative medicine, and tissue engineering. Scientific progress in the field has been steady and expectations for its robust clinical application continue to rise. The pharmacological sciences contribute critically to the accelerated translational progress and clinical utility of regenerative medicine technologies (13). In fact the regenerative pharmacology is "the application of pharmacological sciences to accelerate, optimize, and characterize (either *in vitro or in vivo*) the development, maturation, and function of bioengineered and regenerating tissues."

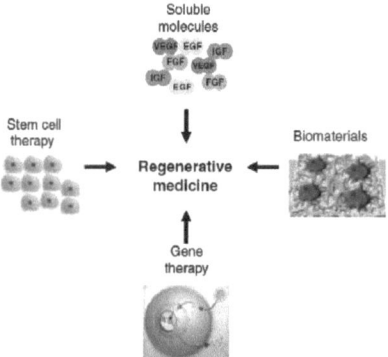

Figure 2: Regenerative medicine is an emerging multidisciplinary field of research and clinical applications focused on the repair, replacement or regeneration of tissue or organs. The approaches may include the use of soluble molecules, gene therapy, stem cell therapy and biomaterials (13).

A particular case is represented by Biobanking, which is a new and dynamic discipline that is being undertaken across a wide range of institutions, both public and private (10). The increasing number of biobanks has helped create networks across institutions and countries, these having developed in order to achieve sufficiently large numbers of tissue samples relating to the same groups of pathologies. Biobanks contain biological samples and associated information that are essential raw materials for advancement of biotechnology, human health, and research and development in life sciences. Population-based and disease-oriented biobanks are major biobank formats to establish the disease relevance of human genes and provide opportunities to elucidate their interaction with environment and lifestyle. The developments in personalized medicine require molecular definition of new disease subentities and biomarkers for identification of relevant patient subgroups for drug development. These emerging demands can only be met if biobanks cooperate at the transnational or even global scale. Establishment of common standards and strategies to cope with the heterogeneous legal and ethical landscape in different countries are seen as major challenges for biobank networks (14). Thanks to international cooperation, these collections are allowing the study of rare types of cancers, as well as tumours that are more common. Several initiatives have been undertaken that aim to organize collection of material with reliable clinical information in order to guarantee high-quality samples adequate for diagnostics, therapy and research. In Europe, more than 225 biobanks and institutions from over 30 countries that collect samples and pathological/clinical data belong to the Biobanking and Biomolecular Resources Research Infrastructure (BBMRI) (15).

4.2 Proteomics

In recent decades, enormous discoveries have been made in the life sciences: among the main results can certainly count the great progress made in sequencing the genomes of the organisms, from prokaryotes to those of eukaryotes. Following a joint effort of the scientific world which knows no equal, in February 2001 was completed the sequence of the human genome: the achievement of this important goal has shifted the attention of researchers towards new projects, targeted to the knowledge of living organisms to a level of greater complexity, which could describe the vital functions in their entirety. The sequencing of the genomes is, in fact, only the starting point for understanding the phenomenon of life, because the meaning of the genetic message of a living organism is divided into different levels of complexity: the immediate, and almost completely described, consists of knowledge of the sequence of individual units of information contained in the itself genome. This information allows, in most cases, to know the messages that preserves genetic information.

The information contained in the genome of an organism is, however, much more complex than the simple sequence of messages deductible from the genomic sequence: every cellular function is the result of the action of protein, real effectors of genetic information. The phenomenon of life is, in its entirety, the result of the interaction of multiple effector proteins, resulting from gene expression, in turn, controlled and mediated by proteins.

Attempts to understand the function that each individual product of expression of a gene in a genome led to the development of techniques and experimental procedures applicable on a large scale that are listed under the name of functional genomics. This area of research includes studies of a different nature from the expression profiles of mRNAs, technology-based DNA chip (16-17) to those of protein. These last are based on two-dimensional electrophoresis and mass spectrometry, up to the definition of the large-scale protein-protein interactions (18) then passing from the field of nucleic acids to the proteins. Just in the context of functional genomics is born proteomics, protein chemistry evolution of the twentieth century, no longer directed to the study of individual proteins but to the entirety of proteins in their functionality, through dynamic events that carry the life cycle (19).

For proteome, a term coined in 1994 by Marc Wilkins, indicating the entire complex of the products of expression of the genome of a cell at a given moment of his life. While the information of a genome is static during the life of an organism, the proteome, in contrast, changes rapidly in response to the many stimuli to which the cell is subjected. This character is so very dynamic and this means that the genomic sequence is necessary but not sufficient to define all the actors of the cell proteins. Therefore, we can affirm that the genome may correspond to a multiple proteomes. We can generally define proteomics as the study of all the proteins of a cell, a tissue, an organ, in terms of expression, post-translational modifications and interactions with other molecules in order to obtain a comprehensive view of the processes cellular protein level.

Depending on the specific objectives can be distinguished from the functional and structural proteomics: the first is aimed at determining the three-dimensional structures of all proteins in an organism, while the second has as its purpose the complete definition of the biological role. The structural proteomics should therefore complement the traditional approaches of structural biology, such as X-ray diffraction and nuclear magnetic resonance spectroscopy to alternative methods such as proteolysis, selective chemical modification, the hydrogen -deuterium exchange, computational chemistry. The functional proteomics has a field of interest even wider: it requires, in fact, a study of the level of expression of proteins and post-translational modifications, cellular localization and protein-protein interaction (20).

4.2.1 Applications in functional proteomics

We can distinguish two main areas of research for functional proteomics: functional proteomics expression proteomics and functional interaction.

The expression proteomics is the study of quantitative changes in the levels of protein expression in cells. Traditionally the experimental procedure most frequently associated to proteomics is the fractionation and separation by two-dimensional electrophoresis, which also allows to quantify the proteins of a proteome and to detect the possible post-translational modifications (21).

The field of interest of functional proteomics is, if possible, even more broadly: the definition of the biological role of the individual elements of the proteome in fact requires an exhaustive study of the level of protein expression and post-translational modifications, cellular localization and protein-protein interactions. In this sense, the study of systems in particular physio-pathological situations and/or in the presence of natural or artificial stimuli, becomes the natural prerequisite for the understanding of the biological role of the components of the "system life."

Fundamental studies of proteomics is to have methods and instruments more accurate and sensitive to identify and quantify proteins. The recent technological development especially in mass spectrometry gave a major boost to research; new technologies now allow the identification of thousands of proteins, making it a realistic possibility to characterize entire proteomes. In fact, there is a growing need to reduce the amount of sample needed and enable the analysis of less abundant protein species, sometimes occurring in a few copies and often involved in important regulatory processes.

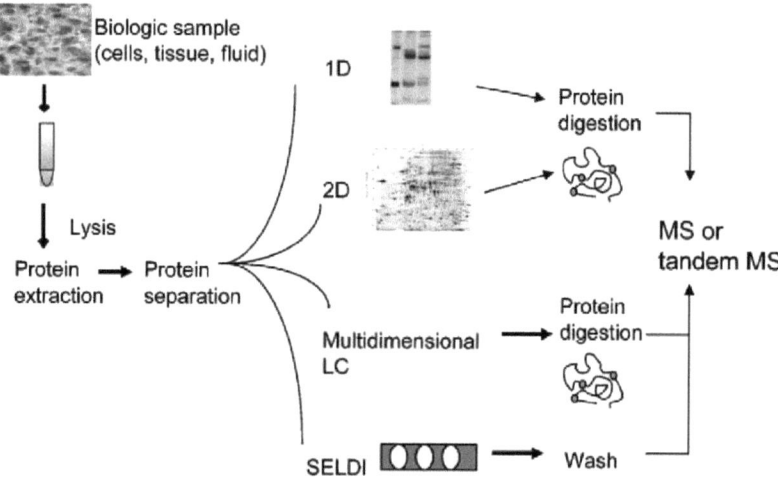

Figure 3: from "Proteomics in pathology research" Overview of experimental design for mass spectrometry-based proteomic studies. Proteins are extracted from biologic samples and fractionated by a variety of separation methods. In 1D gel electrophoresis, proteins are separated by size. In 2D gel electrophoresis, proteins are separated based on isoelectric point (pI) and size. In multidimensional liquid chromatography, digested proteins are fractionated by 2D (strong cationic exchange (SCX) and reverse phase (RP)) or 3D (strong cationic exchange, avidin and reverse-phase) liquid chromatography. In the fourth method, proteins are separated based on functional properties according to physical, chemical or biochemical properties in surface-enhanced laser-desorption ionization (SELDI) technology (22).

4.2.2 Protein Chip

Predictive medicine, utilizing the Protein Chip Array technology, is developed through the implementation of novel biomarkers and multimarker patterns for detecting disease, determining patient prognosis, monitoring drug effects such as efficacy or toxicity, and for defining treatment options. The ProteinChip Array technology is used for the discovery, validation, identification, and characterization of disease-associated proteins from biological samples. The versatile nature of this technology is enabling for a wide variety of applications in both research and clinical proteomics (23).

The novel biomarkers may also serve as novel protein drug candidates or protein drug targets. In addition, this technology can be used for discovering small molecule drugs or for defining their mode of action utilizing protein-based assays. Recent reviews describe applications of the Protein Chip Array technology for discovery and identification of novel inhibitors of HIV-1 replication, serum and tissue proteome analysis for the discovery and development of novel multimarker clinical assays for prostate, breast, ovarian, and other cancers, and biomarker and drug discovery applications for neurological disorders (23, 24).

Numerous cancer-related publications have demonstrated the discovery and development of biomarkers and multimarker patterns for protein-based predictive medicine, but also for drug discovery applications using Alzheimer's disease as the model system (23, 25, 26).

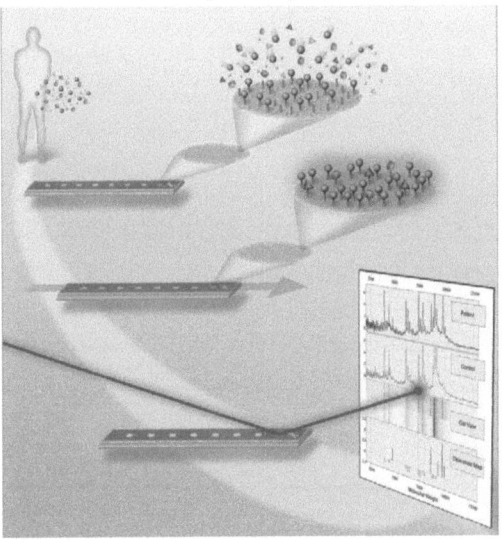

Figure 4: Protein profiling protocol. Procedure for preparing the ProteinChip Arrays with biological samples and for analyzing the retained proteins by SELDI-TOF-MS using a ProteinChip Reader (23).

4.2.3 New biomarkers

Proteomic technologies have experienced major improvements in recent years. Such advances have facilitated the discovery of potential tumor markers with improved sensitivities and specificities for the diagnosis, prognosis and treatment monitoring of cancer patients (6, 27).

Mapping of protein signaling networks within tumors can identify new targets for therapy and provide a means to stratify patients for individualized therapy. Kinases are important drug targets, as such kinase network information could become the basis for development of therapeutic strategies for improving treatment outcome. An urgent clinical goal is to identify functionally important molecular networks associated with subpopulations of patients that may not respond to conventional combination chemotherapy (27, 28).

4.2.4 Stem cells in proteomics

Proteomic methods have produced large data sets of proteins involved in mechanisms and pathways that regulate Stem Cells (SC) proliferation and differentiation. The insights thus obtained in SC biology have also created many opportunities to improve public health. Proteomics may very well contribute to gaining insight into SC functioning and behaviour and thus provide clues for how to tackle these problems. Several important issues, including sample heterogeneity, post-translational modifications, protein-protein interaction, and high-throughput quantification of hydrophobic addressed and require further technical optimization. In fact the various methodologies, used in proteomics, are also used to study SCs, so from sample preparation and protein extraction to two-dimensional electrophoresis and next identification of proteins using Mass Spectrometry, latter is so used for protein profiling and quantitative analysis; without forgetting protein chips and array. Understanding molecular mechanisms underlying SC pluripotency should illuminate fundamental properties of SCs and the process of cellular reprogramming. Proteomics proved to be a powerful approach to gain insight concerning key intracellular signals governing SC self-renewal and differentiation (13, 29).

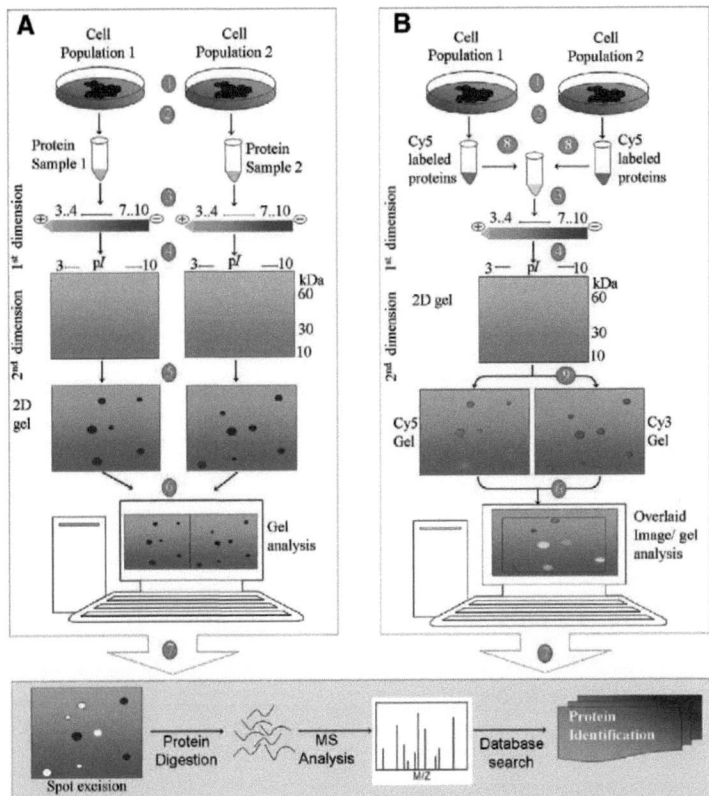

Figure 5: a schematic representation of differential protein display using two-dimensional gel electrophoresis (2-DE) and difference in-gel electrophoresis (DIGE). The number in the center of panel represents the "stage" in the legend. (A): Cell samples are grown under different conditions/treatments (stage I), and total proteins are extracted and subjected to isoelectric focusing (IEF) (first-dimension electrophoresis). The IEF gels are reduced with dithiothreitol and alkylated with iodoacetamide prior to SDS-polyacrylamide gel electrophoresis (SDS-PAGE). The first dimension separates proteins according to isoelectric point (pI), whereas the second dimension separates them approximately according to molecular weight (Mr). Proteins are then visualized using silver, Coomassie Brilliant Blue (CBB), or SYPRO Ruby staining methods, and the protein pattern is captured by a high-resolution camera or densitometer and analyzed by software. The Mr and pI of each protein are estimated by comparison with the mobility of standard proteins, and changes in staining intensity between replicate gels or between treatments are measured. For protein identification, gels are stained with MS-compatible stains such as SYPRO Ruby or CBB. Protein spots are excised from the gel and analyzed by MS. (B): DIGE system includes steps common to 2-DE. However, in DIGE, two protein samples are differentially labeled by Cy3 and Cy5, respectively, and then mixed and run on the same IEF and SDS-PAGE gel. This allows coseparation of different labeled samples in the same gel and ensures that all samples will be subject to exactly the same first- and second-dimension electrophoresis running conditions, limiting experimental variation and resulting in accurate within-gel matching. Following 2D separation, the gel is imaged at the excitation wavelengths of each of fluorescent dye using a scanner, after which an overlay image can be generated. Differences in protein abundance are then accurately quantified using software. Coomassie stain is the most economical and easy-to-use, but having a detection limit of 50–100 ng per spot, it is also the least sensitive. Apart from radioactive gel visualization, silver staining is the most sensitive method, with a detection limit of 1–2 ng. SYPRO Ruby is

very easy to use and almost as sensitive as silver stain, but it is more expensive than CBB and silver staining. Cy3/Cy5 is the most expensive method and requires costly imaging systems, but it shows very small variability with different gels and operators. Unlike silver staining, CBB, SYPRO Ruby, and Cy3/Cy5 show a good compatibility with MS. When the aim of the study is relative quantification between samples, a wide linear dynamic range is required. CBB and silver stain have a low dynamic range (approximately 10-fold), whereas SYPRO Ruby and Cy3/Cy5 represent a much higher dynamic range (1,000-fold) and show better correlation between spot density and protein contentcompared with silver staining (29).

Gene expression analyses of stem cells (SCs) will help to uncover or further define signaling pathways and molecular mechanisms involved in the maintenance of selfrenewal, pluripotency, and/or multipotency. In recent years, proteomic approaches have produced a wealth of data identifying proteins and mechanisms involved in SC proliferation and differentiation.

4.2.5 The Proteomic and the Pathology

During the proteomic era, the 'functional proteomics' has become a powerful tool for unraveling the disease patho-physiology and for biomarker discovery because post-translational modifications such as phosphorylation and glycosylation are very important to identify networks of signaling pathways that are characteristic of physiologic and pathologic states (30-31). Recent studies have applied proteomics for the investigation of several pathology with major aims to search for novel biomarkers and new therapeutic targets. The fundamental applications are:

- diabetic nephropathy, (32)
- diabetic microangiopathy (33)
- human prostate cancer (34)
- neurodegeneration in Alzheimer's disease(35);
- clinical application(36);
- early diagnosis (37).

Diabetic microangiopathy has become a heavy social burden worldwide, but at present it is still difficult to predict and diagnose this ailment at an early stage. Various proteomics approaches have been applied to the pathophysiological study of diabetic microangiopathy. Conventional proteomics methods, including gel-based methods, exhibit limited sensitivity and robustness, have typically used in high- or middle-abundance biomarker discovery. Clinical samples from patients with diabetic microangiopathy, such as biopsy samples, are minute in size. Therefore, sample preparation, quantitative labelling and mass spectrometry technologies need to be optimized for low-abundance protein detection, multiple-sample processing and precision quantitation. Recent technological developments in proteomics tools may shed new light on the pathogenesis of diabetic microangiopathy and biomarkers and therapeutic targets related to this condition.

4.3 Tissue engineering

Tissue engineering is an emerging multidisciplinary and interdisciplinary field involving the development of bioartificial implants and/or the fostering of tissue remodeling with the purpose of repairing or enhancing tissue or organ function. Bioartificial constructs generally consist of cells and biomaterials, so tissue engineering draws from both cell and biomaterials science and technology. Successful applications require a thorough understanding of the environment experienced by cells in normal tissues and by cells in bioartificial devices before and after implantation (38).

In tissue engineering, a highly porous artificial extracellular matrix or scaffold is required to accommodate mammalian cells and guide their growth and tissue regeneration in three dimensions. However, existing three-dimensional scaffolds for tissue engineering proved less than ideal for actual applications, because not only they lack mechanical strength, but they also do not guarantee interconnected channels (39).

In the unites states alone, approximately a quarter of patients in need of organ transplants die while waiting for a suitable donor (40, 41). The current demands for transplant organs and tissues is far outpacing the supply, and all manner of projections indicate that this gap will continue to widen. Cell transplantation as recently been proposed as an alternative treatment to whole organ transplantation for failing or malfunctioning organs. For the creation of an autologous implant, donor tissue is harvested and dissociated into individual cells, and the cells are attached and cultured onto a proper substrate that is ultimately implanted at the desired site of the functioning tissue. Because many isolated cell populations can be expanded *in vitro* using cell culture techniques, only a very small number of donor cells may be necessary to prepare such implants. However, it is believed that isolated cells cannot form new tissues by themselves. Most primary organ cells are believed to be anchorage-dependent and require specific environments that very often include the presence of a supporting material to act as a template for growth. The success of any cell transplantation therapy therefore relies on the development of suitable substrates for both *in vitro* and *in vivo* tissue culture. Currently, these substrates, mainly in the form of tissue engineering scaffolds, prove less than ideal for applications, because not only they lack mechanical strength, but they also suffer from a lack of interconnection channels (42).

4.3.1 Tissue Engineering: From Biology to Biological Substitutes

Hydrogels, microgels and nanogels have emerged as versatile and viable platforms for sustained protein release, targeted drug delivery, and tissue engineering due to excellent biocompatibility, a microporous structure with tunable porosity and pore size, and dimensions spanning from human organs, cells to viruses. In the past decade, remarkable advances in hydrogels, microgels and nanogels have been achieved with click chemistry. It is a most promising strategy to prepare gels with varying dimensions owing to its high reactivity, superb selectivity, and mild reaction conditions. In particular, the recent development of copper-free click chemistry such as strain-promoted azide-alky ne cycloaddition, radical mediated thiol-ene chemistry, Diels–Alder reaction, tetrazole-alkene photo-click chemistry, and oxime reaction renders it possible to form hydrogels, microgels and nanogels without the use of potentially toxic catalysts or immunogenic enzymes that are commonly required. Notably, unlike other chemical approaches, click chemistry owing to its unique bioorthogonal feature does not interfere with encapsulated bioactives such as living cells, proteins and drugs and furthermore allows versatile preparation of micropatterned biomimetic hydrogels, functional microgels and nanogels

The current status and future possibilities, in the development of different bioartificial constructs, including bioartificial skin, cardiovascular implants, bioartificial pancreas, and encapsulated secretory cells. These include, but are not limited to, the development of new cell lines and biomaterials, the evaluation of the optimal construct architecture, and the reproducible manufacture and preservation of bioartificial devices until ready for use (43).

4.3.2 Tissue Engineering: The End of the Beginning

An important factor of translational medicine is impact of current economic conditions. Tissue engineering is very multidisciplinary field but with recent disappointing product launches. Data were collected on all firms known to be active in the field, analyzed, showed more than 2600 full-time equivalents (FTEs) in 15 countries and 89 firms were engaged in tissue-engineering research and development. Annual spending was $487 million, down about 20% since 2000—a reasonable performance in the face of a stagnant economy and difficult capital markets. Individual sectors proved far more volatile. Activity in skin, cartilage, and other structural applications declined by more than 50% with a loss of 800 FTEs. This downsizing was somewhat counterbalanced by a 42% increase in stem cell firms, which added more than 300 employees. Consistent with general disenchantment with technology sector equities, capital value of publicly traded tissue-engineering corporations has decreased by almost 90% from $2.5 billion at the end of 2000 to $300 million at the end of 2002. The United States' fraction of the total workforce declined from 80% in 2000 to 54% in 2002. By the close of 2002, twenty tissue-engineered products had entered Food and Drug Administration clinical trials. Four were approved but none of these are yet commercially successful. Six other applications were either abandoned or failed to achieve product approval. Ten products were still in clinical trials, some of which were investigator sponsored, and most of which were at the phase I/phase II stage. The field has yet to produce a profitable product despite an aggregate research and development investment exceeding $4.5 billion. Tissue engineering is clearly having difficulty transitioning from a development stage industry to one with a successful product portfolio. This is often the case for breakthrough medical technologies (44, 45).

4.3.3 The Growth of Tissue Engineering

At the beginning of 2001, tissue engineering research and development was being pursued by 3,300 scientists and support staff in more than 70 startup companies or business units with a combined annual expenditure of over $600 million. Spending by tissue engineering firms has been growing at a compound annual rate of 16%, and the aggregate investment since 1990 now exceeds $3.5 billion. The net capital value of the 16 publicly traded tissue engineering startups had reached $2.6 billion. Firms focusing on structural applications (skin, cartilage, bone, cardiac prosthesis, and the like) comprise the fastest growing segment. In contrast, efforts in biohybrid organs and other metabolic applications have contracted over the past few years. The number of companies involved in stem cells and regenerative medicine is rapidly increasing, and this area represents the most likely nidus of future growth for tissue engineering. A notable recent trend has been the emergence of a strong commercial activity in tissue engineering outside the United States, with at least 16 European or Australian companies (22% of total) now active (43, 46).

4.3.4 Bone tissue engineering

An important field of research of tissue engineering associated with regenerative medicine is bone tissue engineering. It is "an interdisciplinary field that applies the principles of engineering and the life sciences toward the development of biological substitutes that restore, maintain or improve tissue function". At present, most studies are focused in the development of porous 3D structures, named scaffolds, following the concept of bio-mimicry (literally defined as the imitation of life or nature) to more closely mimic the anatomical and biochemical organization of cells and matrix native to achieve the suitable mechanical properties for the tissue (47, 48). In fact, it is important for tissue engineers to understand the biological events and signals involved, for instance, in musculoskeletal cell and tissue morphogenesis. These signals of bone regeneration are required in large quantity, engineered biomaterials combined with growth factors, such as bone morphogenetic protein-2 (BMP-2), have been demonstrated to be an effective approach in bone tissue engineering, since they can act both as a scaffold and as a drug delivery system to promote bone repair and regeneration. Recent advantages in the field of engineered scaffolds have been obtained from the investigation of composite scaffolds designed by the combination of bioceramics, especially hydroxyapatite (HA), and biodegradable polymers, such as poly (D,L-lactide-coglycolide) (PLGA) and chitosan, in order to realize osteoconductive structures that can mimic the natural properties of bone tissue. This is a classic example of use of different technologies to improve the quality of life, in medicine field. For example, it is demonstrated that the incorporation of growth factors into different composite scaffolds, by encapsulation, absorption or entrapment, could be advantageous in terms of osteo-induction for new bone tissue engineered scaffolds as drug delivery systems and some of them should be further analyzed to optimized the drug release for future therapeutic applications (49, 50).

4.4 Biobanks

Biobanks are central to the process of collection of human biospecimens for translational research and have contributed to numerous advancements in our understanding and treatment of disease (51). Biobanks are collections of human biospecimens (tissues, blood and body fluids and their derivatives collected for diagnosis and/or for research projects) and their associated clinical and outcome data. These biospecimens are typically obtained from a subset of the public who become patients in the health care system. These patients provide biospecimens during clinic visits, diagnostic or therapeutic procedures, or at autopsy. The biospecimens accrued by biobanks are processed and preserved in a variety of ways to support different clinical and research uses, including fixation, freezing and live cell banking. Annotation encompasses documentation of the biospecimen's composition, as well as linkage to health data associated with the patient and their condition, treatment and outcome. Processed and annotated biospecimens are then released to researchers. This typically occurs through selection of biospecimen cohorts from the biobank database using specified criteria to allow a specific research question to be addressed (51, 52).

The Central Research Infrastructure for Molecular Pathology (CRIP), the concept for a pan-European Biobanking and Biomolecular Resources Research Infrastructure (BBMRI), and the Organization for Economic Co-operation and Development (OECD) global Biological Resources Centres network are examples for transnational, European and global biobank networks .

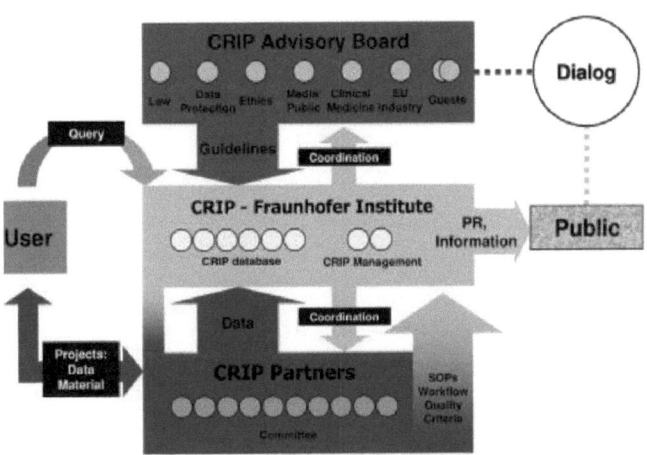

Figure 6: Structure and organization of CRIP. Users send their queries to the CRIP database on whether samples and data required for a specific research project are available at CRIP partner institutions. Users and CRIP partners then agree on the research projects. The CRIP management may provide administrative support for project execution. The Advisory Board provides guidelines for the strategy and operation of CRIP and supports the management in communication with the scientific community and general public (52).

4.5 Conclusions

In a world that creates more figures super specialized, translational medicine is the way to return to have an overview of the medical problems, but starting just from a scientific research strongly finalized. We can conclude, as a result of wheeled of information, in this chapter, that the goal is to improve human health and thus to contribute to translational research. Starting from the studies of the biology up, until the tessue engeeinerign, passing through proteomics, with all the shades, as the functional, or that of the stem cells, and again through the creation of biobanks, all these disciplines can be seen as branches of medicine. In fact through translational research, in the various fields of research, are fundamental to the advancement of translational medicine and to allow to find new solutions to help, to understand or to create new molecular target for pathologies also very different.

Only the scientific progress, not detached from the real medical problems, will allow real progress and then the emergence of translational medicine.

Fundamental role is represented by stackholders, public and private, such as universities and pharmaceutical companies, which should help scientific research to advance toward a search, not an end in itself, but a real solution, through dialogue and the continual exchange of information between scientists, doctors, nurses and patients.

References

1. Littman BH, DI Mario L, Plebani M and Marincola FM. What's next in translational medicine? Clinical Science (2007) 112, 217–227
2. Mankoff SP, Brander C, Ferrone S and Marincola FM. Lost in translation: obstacles to translational medicine. J. Transl. Med. (2004) 2, 14
3. Szalma S, Koka V, Khasanova T, Perakslis ED et al. Effective knowledge management in translational medicine. Journal of Translational Medicine (2010,) 8: 68
4. Lehmann F, Lacombe D, Therasse P, Eggermont AM. Integration of Translational Research in the European Organization for Research and Treatment of Cancer Research (EORTC). Clinical Trial Cooperative Group Mechanisms. J Transl Med. (2003) 7;1(1): 2
5. Ferrari M. Cancer nanotechnology: opportunities and challenges Nat Rev Cancer. (2005) 5(3):161-71

6. Fakruddin MD, Hossain Z. and Afroz H. Prospects and applications of nanobiotechnology: a medical perspective. Journal of Nanobiotechnology (2012), 10:31

7. Weston AD, Hood L Systems Biology, Proteomics, and the Future of Health Care: Toward Predictive, Preventative, and Personalized Medicine, Journal of Proteome Research 2004, 3, 179-196

8. Zoon KC, Kohn EC, Barrett JC, Liotta LA, Petricoin EF. Clinical proteomics: translating benchside promise into bedside reality, Nat Rev Drug Discov. (2002) 1(9):683-95.

9. Paulo JA, Kadiyala V, Banks PA, SteenH, ConwellDL, Mass Spectrometry-Based Proteomics for Translational Research: A Technical Overview Journal of biology and medicine (2012), 85:59-73

10. Chaurand P, Sanders ME, Jensen RA, Caprioli RM.. Proteomics in diagnostic pathology: profiling and imaging proteins directly in tissue sections. Am J Pathol. (2004) ;165(4):1057-1068

11. Zhu H, Qian J. Applications of Functional Protein Microarrays in Basic and Clinical Research, Adv Genet. (2012) 79: 123–155

12. Zhu H, Cox E, Qian J. Functional protein microarray as molecular decathlete: aversatile player in clinical proteomics. Proteomics Clin Appl. (2012) 6(11-12):548-62

13. Dieckmann C, Renner R, Milkova L, and Jan C. Regenerative medicine in dermatology: biomaterials, tissue engineering, stem cells, gene transfer and beyond. Exp Dermatol. (2010) 19(8):697-706.

14. Botti G, Franco R, Cantile M, Ciliberto G and Ascierto PA Tumor biobanks in translational medicine Journal of Translational Medicine (2012) 10:204

15. Asslaber M, Zatloukal K. Biobanks: translational, European and global networks. Brief Funct Genomic Proteomic (2007) 6:193–201

16. Schena M, Shalon D, Davis RW, Brown PO; Quantitative monitoring of gene expression patterns with a complementary DNA microarray. Science (1995) 270, 467-470

17. Brown PO, Botstein D. Exploring the new world of the genome with DNA microarrays. Nat. Genet. (1999). 21, 33-37

18. Uetz P, Giot L, Cagney G, Mansfield TA, Judson RS, Knight JR, Lockshon D, Narayan V Sinivasan M, Pochart P, Qureshi-Emili A, Li Y, Godwin B, Conover D, Kalbfleisch T, Vijayadamodar G, Yang M, Johnston M, Fields S, Rothberg JM. A comprehensive analysis of

protein-protein interactions in *Saccharomyces cerevisiae*. Nature (2000) 403, 623-627

19.Tyers M, Mann M. From genomics to proteomics. Nature (2003) 422, 193-197

20.Zimmermann JD, Brown LR. Perspectives for mass spectrometry and functional proteomics. Mass Spectrom. Rev. (2001) 20, 1-57

21.Anderson NG, Anderson NL. Twenty years of two-dimensional electrophoresis: past, present and future. Electrophoresis (1996) 17, 443-453

22.Megan SL, Kojo SJ, Elenitoba J. Proteomics in pathology research. Laboratory Investigation (2004) 84, 1227–1244

23.Reddy G and Dalmasso EA. SELDI ProteinChip Array Technology: Protein-Based Predictive Medicine and Drug Discover.y Applications Journal of Biomedicine and Biotechnology (2003) 237–241

24.Zhu H, Cox E, Qian J. The Functional Protein Microarray Molecular Decathlete: A Versatile Player in Clinical Proteomics, Proteomics Clin Appl. (2012); 6(0): 548–562

25.Uzoma I, Zhu H. Interactome Mapping: Using Protein Microarray Technology to Reconstruct Diverse Protein Networks. Genomics Proteomics Bioinformatics 11 (2013) 18–28

26.Seibert V, Ebert MP, Buschmann T. Advances in clinical cancer proteomics: SELDI-ToF-mass spectrometry and biomarker discovery. Brief Funct Genomic Proteomic (2005) 4(1): 16–26

27.Martino TA, Tata N, Bjarnason GA, Straume M, Sole MJ. Diurnal protein expression in blood revealed by high throughput mass spectrometry proteomics and implications for translational medicine and body time of day. Am J Physiol Regul Integr Comp Physiol (2007) 293: 1430–1437

28.Levin A, Lancashire W, Fassett RG. Targets, trends, excesses, and deficiencies: refocusing clinical investigation to improve patient outcomes. Outcomes Kidney Int. (2013) 83(6): 1001-109.

29.Baharvand H, Fathi A, Van hoof D, Salekdehd GH. Concise Review: Trends in Stem Cell Proteomics STEMCELLS (2007) 25:1888–1903

30.McLafferty FW, Breuker K, Jin M, Han X, Infusini G, Jiang H, Kong X and Tadhg P. Begley Top-down MS, a powerful complement to the high capabilities of proteolysis proteomics FEBS Journal 274 (2007) 6256–6268

31.Perez OD, Nolan GP. Phospho-proteomic immune analysis by flow cytometry: from mechanism to translational medicine at the single-cell level. Immunol Rev. (2006) 210: 208-228.

32.Thongboonkerd V. Study of diabetic nephropathy in the proteomic era. Proteomic Era Contrib Nephrol. (2011) 170: 172–183

33.Ma Y, Yang C, Tao Y, Zhou H, Wang Y. Recent technological developments in proteomics shed new light on translational research on diabetic microangiopathy FEBS Journal 280 (2013) 5668–5681

34.Petricoin EF, Ornstein DK, Paweletz CP, Ardekani A, et al. Serum Proteomic Patterns for Detection of Prostate Cancer. Journal of the National Cancer Institute, (2002) 94, 16-2,

35.Johnson MD(1), Yu LR, Conrads TP, Kinoshita Y, Uo T, McBee JK, Veenstra TD, Morrison RS The proteomics of neurodegeneration. Am J Pharmacogenomics. (2005) 5(4): 259-70.

36.Colantonio DA, Chan DW. The clinical application of proteomics. Clinica Chimica Acta (2005) 357(2)24: 151–158,

37.Diamandis EP. Analysis of serum proteomic patterns for early cancer diagnosis: drawing attention to potential problems. J Natl Cancer Inst. (2004) 96(5): 353-356

38.Romagnoli C, D'Asta F, Brandi ML. Drug delivery using composite scaffolds in the context of bone tissue engineering. Clinical Cases in Mineral and Bone Metabolism (2013) 10(3): 155-161

39.Blum HE. Advances in individualized and regenerative medicine Advances in Medical Sciences 59 (2014) 7–12

40.U.S. Scientific Registry for Organ Transplantation and the Organ Procurement and Transplant Network. Annual Report. Richmond VA: UNOS, 1990.

41.Vacanti J, and Vacanti C. The challenge of tissue engineering. In: Lanza, R.P., Langer, R., and Chick, W.L., eds. Principles of Tissue Engineering. Austin, TX: Academic Press, 1997, pp. 1–6.

42.Yang S, Leong K, Du Z, Chua C, Liebert MA. The Design of Scaffolds for Use in Tissue Engineering. Part I. Traditional Factors Review Tissue Engineering (2001) 7, (6): 679-689

43.Nerem RM. And Schuttle S. The Challenge of Imitating Nature. Principles of Tissue Engineering, 3rd Edition (2007) Chapter 2

44.Nerem RM, Regenerative medicine: the emergence of an industry J. R. Soc. Interface (2010) 7, 771-775

45.Vacanti J and Vacanti CA The History and Scope of Tissue Engineering. Principles of Tissue Engineering (Book) 3rd Edition (2007) Chapter 1

46.Lysaght MJ, Jaklene CA, Deweerd E. Great Expectations: Private Sector Activity in Tissue Engineering, Regenerative Medicine, and Stem Cell Therapeutics TISSUE ENGINEERING: (2008) Part A: 14, (2): 305-317

47.Ma PX. Biomimetic materials for tissue engineering. Advanced Drug Delivery Reviews (2008) 60, 2: 184–198

48.Tabata Y. Biomaterial technology for tissue engineering applications J. R. Soc. Interface (2009) 6, 311–324

49.Makowski MR, Botnar RM. MR imaging of the arterial vessel wall: molecular imaging from bench to bedside. Radiology. (2013) 269:34-51

50.Sah RL, Ratcliffe A. Translational models for musculoskeletal tissue engineering and regenerative medicine. Tissue Eng Part B Rev. (2010) 16(1):1-3

51.Watson PH, Wilson-McManus JE, Barnes RO, et al. Evolutionary concepts in biobanking - the BC J Transl Med. (2009) 12;7:95.

52.Asslaber M and Zatloukal K, Biobanks: transnational, European and global networks. Briefings in functional genomics and proteomics. (2007) 6: 193-201

Books!

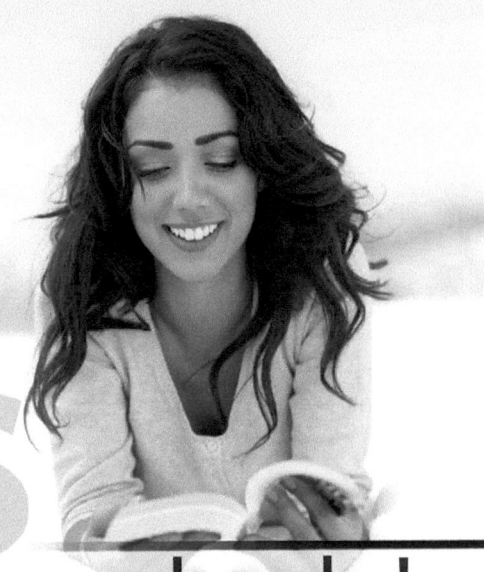

yes

I want morebooks!

Buy your books fast and straightforward online - at one of the world's fastest growing online book stores! Environmentally sound due to Print-on-Demand technologies.

Buy your books online at

www.get-morebooks.com

Kaufen Sie Ihre Bücher schnell und unkompliziert online – auf einer der am schnellsten wachsenden Buchhandelsplattformen weltweit!
Dank Print-On-Demand umwelt- und ressourcenschonend produziert.

Bücher schneller online kaufen

www.morebooks.de

OmniScriptum Marketing DEU GmbH
Heinrich-Böcking-Str. 6-8
D - 66121 Saarbrücken
Telefax: +49 681 93 81 567-9

info@omniscriptum.com
www.omniscriptum.com

OMNIScriptum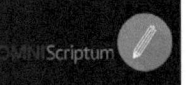

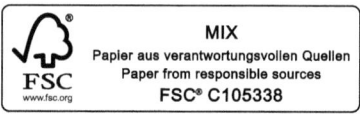

MIX
Papier aus verantwortungsvollen Quellen
Paper from responsible sources
FSC® C105338

FSC
www.fsc.org

Printed by Books on Demand GmbH, Norderstedt / Germany